THE
AMERICAN HERBAL APOTHECARY BIBLE

3-in-1

The Best Herbalism Encyclopedia, Herbal Dispensatory and Herbal Remedies & Recipes to Heal and Improve your Wellness With the Native Americans Spiritual Traditions

Aiyana Henhawk

Table of Contents

NATIVE AMERICAN HERBALISM ENCYCLOPEDIA

The forgotten secrets of medicinal plants & their uses for healing. Eradicate All Diseases From Your Body and Mind Without Side Effects.

Introduction

For generations before the arrival of Europeans in the Modern World, Native Americans studied TM. The health beliefs of this period of time are not familiar, because the archaeological documents are difficult to interpret, and oral histories lack the breadth of time required. Skeletal documentation in some instances suggests head binding, trephination, teeth removal, and other procedures culminating in bone modification, but it is difficult to discover their cultural meaning. The skeletal study, of course, may offer further detail, but predominant American Indians & Alaska Natives might be hesitant to allow researchers to investigate dead ancestors, & they have the right to do so under the statute.

Instead of experimental research, the Native American Graves Safety & Repatriation Act (NAGPRA), passed in 1990, agreed to rebury uncovered ancestral remains and related burial goods. More knowledge of TM can be found in communication cycles and later documents, now prized by tribal communities trying to recreate early traditions, in comparison to the scant details from prehistoric times. Early historical sources, for instance, talk of Aleut's wound care abilities, including washing and suturing puncture wounds with sinew thread & bone needles. Outsiders welcomed this example of medical experience, but a great deal of indigenous information was devalued, and the encounter era took an enormous toll on Native Americans & their communities.

This book will cover all the details about the common herbs and their usage in daily life and common diseases. So wait no more and dive into this beautiful world of herbalism and learn all about the different techniques of harvesting herbs in your backyard.

Fundamentals of Native American Herbalism and How to Grow and Treat Them

The Native American healing practices go back several years since the different tribal communities of North America learned that by mixing roots, spices, and other naturally occurring plants, they could cure numerous medical problems. Yet treatments for Native Americans alone were not part of the healing method.

Healing practices ranged from one group to another tribe, involving numerous gatherings, rituals, and different knowledge of healing, including North America's more than 2,000 indigenous groups. While there were no absolute curing requirements, most tribes accepted that wellness was the manifestation of the spirit and a constant method of remaining strong emotionally, psychologically, and mentally. This power would hold sickness and harm away, preserving harmony with oneself, others nearest to them, the natural world, and the Maker as well. Each person was liable for their welfare, and all perceptions & behaviors had effects, like disabilities, bad luck, illness, or trauma. And when unity was rightly established could their wellbeing be restored.

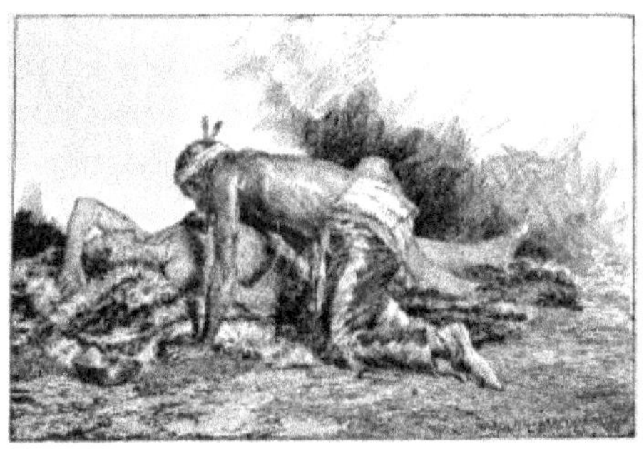

Herbal treatments play an important role in these medicinal rituals, extending further away from the symptoms and aches of the body and beyond the domain of peace and faith. The plants and other natural items used in medicines are obtained from their environment in general, resulting in a further variety of cures. Locally inaccessible goods were, however, also traded over long distances. It was often considered that medicinal plants & herbs were extremely holy. Many different activities have been communicated orally and never reported in writing from one generation to another one, making many curing solutions a mystery. The healers, including the Cherokee, who developed a written language, seldom put their methods or formulas in writing.

They were surprised to see Native Americans suffering from infections and illnesses that they believed were fatal following the advent of early Europeans in the U.S. 500

years earlier. The medicinal medicines of the Indians were much superior to those common to the immigrants in many ways. Yet for the Native Americans, who will wipe out all of them during the next few years, they had no remedies for the "civilization diseases," or the diseases of white men, such as measles and smallpox. These numerous Native Americans, and wisdom that went to the grave with healers, were destroyed. Mostly, despite missing some of the knowledge, it has persisted to this day, used by both Native Americans and non-natives alike. Several contemporary medications rely on herbs & plants that have been used for years by Indians. There are still more than two hundred botanicals in use in pharmaceuticals initially extracted from Native Americans.

As Western colonialism brought new environments to Americans of European origin, as well as the subsequent injuries and diseases in the 1800s, indigenous cultures often supplied the colonists and settlers with herbal medicines that proved necessary for their survival. Any of our great explorers, fur trappers, surgeons, and writings by naturalists, such as Meriwether Lewis & William Clark, Jedediah Strong Smith, Peter Kalm, Leonard McPhail, & William Bartram, include references to the knowledge and use of these plants by native food and medicinal plants obtained from American Indians for the treatment of illness and injury. Miners subsisted during the California

Gold Rush on meals of bacon, peanuts, and coffee. Thus, showing symptoms of scurvy, the foothill tribes (Sierra Nevada), an edible herb that restores fitness, introduced them to Claytonia perfoliata. During the Civil War, local plants such as dogwood (Cornus spp.), sassafras (Sassafras albidum), white oak leaves & bark (Quercus alba), partridgeberry (Mitchella repens), and Liriodendron tulipifera (tulip trees) equipped field surgeons with a repertoire of drugs for the care of wounded soldiers. Eventually, this plant was determined to be rich in Vitamin C and was named 'miner's lettuce.

Immigrants from Europe to the new world do not depend exclusively on Native American herbal medicine. They brought seeds & cutting of favored medicinal plants with them, beneficiaries of Europe's rich herbalist tradition, and unfamiliar with the characteristics of plants common to the Western World. They used Euphrasia Officinalis (eyebright) by Marrubium vulgare (horehound) to relieve inflamed skin, handled colds & coughs, and used Hypericum perforatum (St. John's wort) as an anti-inflammatory. It was this knowledge of the therapeutic characteristics of plants that inspired them to follow Indian herbal data and to quickly incorporate the native plants they read about into their medicine cabinets.

As the Old World organisms brought to the coasts of America, both knowingly and accidentally, rapidly spread to create numerous biological mixtures throughout new world ecosystems, so did medicinal herbs of both local and European roots combine together in the pharmacopeias of the young country. Nearly half of the substances utilized by native plants were used by American Indians, such as Canadian fleabane (Leptilon canadense now Conyza canadensis) and American senna, in the first Pharmacopeia (U.S.) issued in 1820 (Cassia marilandica and Senna marilandica). The equilibrium was made up of non-native plants taken from the homelands of old European or other continents.

Therefore, Americans had exposure to a very wide range of medicinal herbs from the flora of two continents in the early years of our nation, one going back millennia, representing the mutual history of two different herbal societies. However, for American Indians, this mixing approach had one unfortunate feature: their contributions to this extensive collection of medicines were largely forgotten and ignored. To the present day, the oversight persists. In the United States, more than 200 medicines used by American Indians have been or are now mentioned. Pharmacopeia or National Form, but this fact is not recognized by any guide. The tremendous benefits we have gained from the conventional knowledge with natural herbal remedies are still completely uncredited.

1.1Foraging and Reaping

Cultivating your own herbs at home is an enjoyable way to taste fresh flavors all year long. And as the weather starts becoming cooler and the days get shorter, there's just one thing that means: harvest season.

There are a few things you can keep in mind when cultivating plants, no matter what herb you're picking. Here's a tip that is realistic:

- Just pick herbs when they're dry. It is advisable to reap after the morning dew has gone, or at night.

- Just before the opening of the buds should you harvest culinary herbs. Be sure to pinch several buds before they open, since after they flower, all the plant's energy goes into developing blooms, and then the tasty leaves do not grow well.

- Harvest the seeds until they turn from green to brown. The seeds have to be fragile, dry, and crushable, not brown, but brown.

- Be gentle. Handle them carefully to stop bruising your precious crop when harvesting, as fresh herbs are fragile, so.

Sustainable Foraging Recommendations

1. The abundant plants with a broad, scattered population are forage only.

Not extracting a plant and the threats it may pose from commercial demand or loss of habitat after first assessing the population. For e.g., a plant may be geographically abundant, but if there is a universal ultimatum, it may easily disappear, with overharvesting decimating the population.

2. Favor for harvesting non-native species.

If the herb is native and connected to local food chains or is a deserter from another location is among the first things we remember when choosing which herbs to eat. Through competing with them for natural resources, nonnatives relocate native animals. With the same balances and checks that natural plants have encountered, these resourceful plants have not grown nearby, and so they often thrive. This brands them as primary forage for us humans, especially because they remain close to places we live, thriving in neighborhoods, gardens, fields, & the like. Non-natives include Rosa multiflora (multiflora rose), Lonicera japonica (Japanese honeysuckle), Albizia julibrissin (Mimosa), Arctium minus (burdock), and several species of raspberry and blackberry are some of our most popular wild feeble medicinal items in the United States (southeast) (Rubus spp).

3. Tend the gaps "in between".

Wild weeds will naturally arise & make themselves at home with those of you who cultivate a greenhouse and cohabit comfortably with developed vegetables and herbs. You can use plenty of techniques to make them play fair, and you can collect still more medication and food from your greenhouse as an opportunity to serve as a botanical referee! This is the bounty that develops between the medicines and vegetables you have not created yet, that you still have to reap. Frank Cook, a plant friend who died, used to teach in classes that in the form of useful opportunistic plants, more than half of the abundance of a garden may be found in the "in-between." People around the world profit from this vast resource, casually "cultivating" weeds in the regions in between.

Let us take the quarters of the lamb as an example of this form of useful-weed-&-planted-crop-polyculture. More protein, beta-carotene, vitamin C, zinc, and calcium than cultivated spinach are given by lamb parts, often called wild spinach. Why will you root out such a strong plant that does not need special treatment or protection from pests to make way for crops that are less stable and more difficult to develop? You should leave the wild spinach in the field between the newly planted vegetables and the herbal crops. The vegetables fill up after planting the wild spinach for a few weeks or a month, and then you can take out the lamb quarters and use them as mulch for the cultivated crops. Because it makes its way into the greenhouse, wild spinach needs little planting and is relatively disease-free and insect-free.

4. Be a steward purely.

And when you pick sufficiently (possibly pesky) species, adhere to a code of ethics. You deal for, after all, real, breathing animals. Take what you need, leave the beauty of the wake (leave no trace) and make a bid before you go, to make a poem, a little water, hair, a handful of grain. An offering demands a sense of appreciation, reciprocity, and respect.

If you are more science-minded, you might take a minute to consciously relax, meditating on the reciprocity of the exchange of plant-human oxygen, cellular respiration, & photosynthesis. At first, you can sound ridiculous, but give yourself the chance to be shocked. This is how the ancient plant-human dance of friendly friendship, touch, & love influences us.

Be very careful not to overharvest if the plant you are harvesting is organic, so you have already assessed that it is plentiful enough to produce. If you are picking a multi-stem herbaceous plant, cut out a stem or two from each plant. Scatter the crop around a wider field and ensure sure you leave plants with enough flowers and fruit to reproduce. Replant the root crown while you are extracting roots or take only part of the root system of each plant.

Be careful to cut back the aboveground portions while digging up roots so that the plant does not get saturated by water with a root structure that no longer suits its aboveground growth. For resistant weeds with global dispersion, Ses' regenerative methods do not even need to be pursued.

5. Harvesting in situations where you realize that no one has applied herbicide.

Since the surrounding soil is typically polluted with lead, herbicides, and other toxins, there should be no planting of plants near highways, railroads, and power lines. Typically, farm at least 30 feet from the road and ensure sure you do not farm in an environmentally sensitive area (such as a dirty river flood bank). And with herbicides, hay fields can be added.

The foundations are often troublesome in older buildings and they are usually sprayed for pest protection or weeds. Consider visiting a nearby organic urban farm or community garden if you reside in an environment where you can find a number of tasty vegetables, along with gardeners who are eager to share the harvest.

1.2Wildcrafting

Wildcrafting is the ancient art of harvesting untouched, natural growth areas of herbs and plants. Make sure you have permission to select and that normal outdoor security procedures are observed. When you harvest in the near future, make sure to take just what you will need; this will allow for enough growth in exchange for your next visit.

It is necessary that it be carried out with reverence and consciousness when one enters the world and the plants to obtain drugs. People who receive medicine in a religious way from indigenous cultures have done so in identical ways around the globe. The behavioral patterns that underlie them remain the same, although some of the strategies can vary. It is only when plants are used as resources that they continue to be cultivated without thinking. It can take months or even years to gain an appreciation of what you see when you walk into the plant environment. There is a world of complex interrelationships that we do not readily appreciate since we have been disconnected from it for too long. It is necessary to remember that comprehension needs time and that you are a beginner. Natawika, "Thinking like a mountain" is probably the most important attitude to remember. This term is from A Sand County Almanac by Aldo Leopold. Think like a hill, "think like a mountain," He and a friend were having lunch at the moment and saw what they thought was a deer swimming in the lake beneath them. They knew it was a wolf when the deer eventually hit the bank and crawled back. The mother's wolf was briefly joined in joyful abandon by her litter. Leopold & his buddy fired their guns into them round after round. They all thought that less wolves meant a guy could destroy more deer. When they were done, the mother and one cub were mortally wounded, and the others survived. Leopold noted: "Leopold noted:" I realized then, and have also known ever since, that in those eyes there was something new to me, something only known to her and the mountains. The central aspect of researching medicine and harvesting seeds is this mindset and awareness. With the experience of just ten species, the majority of infectious diseases may be treated. Some opioid consumers may know as little as one or two or three or may know as many as a thousand or four, but ten is always appropriate. Thc plants that grow from far away do not need to be known; those that establish near you, in the back yard or in gardens near your house, have all the healing power available. There, nice, really. You both function and are part of the same ecosystem in the same area. The same water is exchanged with you and the same environment. You belong to the same group. You begin to interact with the land on which you live when you start with these popular plants. Year after year, you'll see and pick the same species, from the same stands and from the same area. Your awareness of the medicinal importance of these plants will widen every year. Lots of details regarding them can be learned. The potential to evoke their soothing power would also grow as well. In each plant community from which the plant population has come, grandfather & grandmother plants live. It is important to keep these plants intact. They live & seed down at the peak of the hills as well. They may be truly ancient, thousands of years ago. They look to the unschooled eye much like many others. There were several of these plants here as the boundless sheets of ice retreated north. In this planet, they have seen mankind take their first measures. One plant of chaparral in the southwest desert has also been carbon-dated to be 12,000 years of age. 5 Others are much older. In the middle of a certain era and experience, you can arrive humbly. His grandparents and his grandmother's plants should be left undisturbed. They need to be celebrated with tobacco & smudge, prayer, & celebration. When you encounter that one, you meet the archetypal of its kind, and it has immense power. Behind the old ones are the newer plants and their kin. Food and medications need to be handled like these. Prayers and the selling of tobacco. It would more often lead the plant to die as a consequence if you chose the root. It offers its life love and takes this into account for your need. Some plants, including OSHA, have really long roots, and it's hard to get a whole root. Here, this is a positive idea. When the root falls off, in the next year or even the year after that, still in the field, the remainder may continue to spread and grow a new above-ground vine. Other plants are not this way, and the actual plant is destroyed by root digging. For this purpose, many people assume that only after seeding in the fall and when the strength of the plant begins to go down below the stage will root be collected. However, those roots are more potent when dug in season, and now is probably the time to dig them. While most people assume that plants are inactive in winter, the roots are already developing all the time, when all the stored energy is used to generate the new plant and seeds, which are finally accumulated for spring. In spring, several roots would be fatter and more essential. It is the case with OSHA. When you harvest plants on time, you will come to recognize which plants are better grown in spring and in fall. Other roots, such as those of the red root, are stronger in the fall after the first heavy freeze (Ceanothus Americanus). The inner bark of the root reaches a brilliant red tint, and a pinkish tinge spreads across the white root itself occasionally. The root lotion or tea is deeply red in color, and it is way stronger when derived from fall roots. Most roots can be drained from the heat in a well-aerated position. Looking at them every day, feeling them, and keeping close communication between yourself and the heart is vital. When you develop a root, replace the soil in the hole you have created. Spread the seeds if the seed is in the plant. When you pull up the stems, shake the dirt out of your hand or knee. See and observe the source. Its okay, is it? A strong sense of toughness and a lack of rot or mold should be provided to the source. There are a couple of roots which need cleaning. The coralroot (Corallorhiza maculata) is one example. The white coral-like root is so mixed with the rich soil that the easily broken root is almost impossible to isolate from the earth without washing it in a colander. People sometimes loop smaller roots and hang them to dry. Larger roots need to be split in two to avoid mold and to encourage drying. Drying up roots that are quite mucilaginous and moist requires even longer than other, dryer roots. If a two-year plant is a root that you cultivate, in the fall of the first year or the spring of the second year, harvest the root. Usually, roots can survive many years before losing viability, although it differs with each plant. Touch them and enjoy their beauty until you cut them if you pick the leaves and stems from the above-ground parts of a plant. The best time to select them is in the early morning because they are still fresh with dew and before the sun has wilted them. In order to avoid mold, whether you are attempting to dry them, bind the leaves together in a bundle not much wider than an inch long. In a sunny, well-ventilated place, hang them from the light, top-down. Up to next year, make sure you quit the roots and come back with fresh seeds. Know that the above-ground parts of the vine, such as goldenseal and American ginseng, are as productive as the roots of other goods. The leaf content is not collected and marketed in factories since it does not stand up in factories. Leafy plants need not be sprayed, just shaken and easily washed by hand before drying. If there are bugs in them, shake them off vigorously. Overground plants will only live for a year before losing productivity. Generally, they ought to be replaced next year. In the fall, barks are best chosen, although at some periods of the year they do not come off the log as easily as others. I like chopping the leaves and leaving all the trees to begin growing. The bark should be stripped off the branch just before it has a chance to settle. To dry out from the humidity, it should be in a well-ventilated location. A few barks, though, profit, like white willow, from a few hours of drying in clear sunlight.

The fragrance of the willow, so clearly a part of the plant and its medicine, becomes much stronger when enabled to appreciate the sunlight for a moment. Pay attention to where you pick seeds. Make careful note to carry with you so many of the trees. Some plants, such as coralroot, are very rare in scale, and about one in every four visible plants can be extracted. Pay attention to your thoughts and medicine, and take only what you need. Ask the plants how many of them you can afford. Even then, take attention. Pay heed, too, to where you are choosing plants. In certain days and times, the soil is still sick, and so are the plants that grow there. Whole plants lose potency much more steadily than broken or powdered plants. Hold the crops as full as practicable. Store them as far from the sun and air as possible. It has been popular in many cultures to hang plants in the rafters of lodges and houses and use them all winter and then cover them the next year. The capacity to excavate medication is a trained and coordinated ability. There are tons of stuff to learn and plenty of abilities to create. Many individuals do so in various forms. It is a craft like woodworking or leatherworking. You recall thoughts with the heart, you remember the soul with the spirit, and you remember the particulars of searching with the mind. When her mother stuck a needle into the lobe of one of her ears when she was inattentive, her mother decided to show her the usage of plants when she was a girl. "She persisted carelessly, and her mother pierced the other ear, saying, "This will make you listen to what I think." Her mother instructed her to try to recall the herbs and their uses, saying, "A sick individual who is not saved by a doctor may come to you sometime after I'm dead and ask for Natawika's remedies." Realizing the value attached to obtaining pay for services by her mother, Harri If the set was extended over a wider region and consumed a longer period of time, it would have collected a significantly larger number.

Some of the suggestions regarding wildcrafting are as follows.

1. Don't ever collect animals that are in distress or threatened. At the closest herbarium or botanical garden, check the catalog of these species. You may also contact the American Guild of Herbalists for a nationwide listing.

2. For authentication, use keys and specimens with vouchers.

3. Ask for permission and give thanks, note all bonds in life, express your appreciation.

4. To sow downslope-grandparent plants, leave mature & seed-producing plants within the stand and at the hilltop. Work the way up.

5. If unclear, extract no more than ten percent of the whole native plant and root and thirty percent of the native species of naturalized plants or flowers and leaves. Collecting only from abundant stands. Harvest conservatively to ensure the maintenance and well-being of plant species.

1.3Strategies to Expand and Spread

1. Using proper wildcraft techniques will ensure reduced effects, increase crop yields, and help provide plant food for wildlife. Do not harvest the same stand year after year, but tend the field as needed. Thinning, root splitting, top pinching, and defense of a large range of grandparent plants are methods used for 'gardening' to seed and protect young plants.2. Be conscious of factors that lead to erosion. If you dig roots and close holes, replant or scatter seeds. Be mindful of hillside stands and install foliage and soil around cleared areas. Collecting leaves from nearby harvested plants and spreading it around maybe fit. Wearing hard-soled shoes will infect vulnerable hillside habitats with irreparable damage.

3. Do not pull the roots when the leaves are being removed. By flower pruning of certain varieties, root yields, as well as foliage, may be increased.

4. Enable seasonal results for wildlife-generated areas. Be aware of your harvested stands and monitor the different growth cycles. This will calculate the real environmental effects. (An existing wild crafter in the northwest has learned that once it reaches stasis, a healthy population can grow by around 30 percent a year. Something less than this can be considered degenerative.)

1.4Suggested Gathering Times

1. Aerial or above ground constituents: 6 a.m. - 10 a.m. In the morning, before they are wilting in the sun. Some are better when harvesting leaves only prior to flowering.

You should be able to see the color of the bud by only choosing most flowers until they begin to bloom. The standard moon cycle for gathering aerial pieces is before or after the full moon.

2. Roots: early in the morning or before sunrise harvest after seeding, if necessary. Biennials: harvest in the fall of the first year or season of the second year. A traditional time is a new moon.

3. Barks: Harvest during spring or fall. Don't necessarily strip. Grab a whole crop. Tree thinning is appropriate in dense cities, but the healthiest looking trees refuse to leave. If you take only from the tiny leaves, be careful of possibly making the tree susceptible to fungal rot. The inner bark, or cambium, for pollarding, is the most involved bark among many, leaving small trunks and low stumps for copping. This will have continuous production. Three-quarters of the waning light is the traditional bark method.

4. Saps and Pitches: Harvest in late winter or early spring.

5. Crop and Fruit: Harvest with some differences when mature, such as bananas, unripe pods of scarlet beans, etc.

1.5Drying Out

1. Dry most plants; stop wire screens and newspaper printing in shaded, well-ventilated regions. Analysis into which plants in the sundry better.

2. Don't wash the trees or bulbs. To clean off rodents and dust, shake them. Where quantities are appropriate, attach bundles at the stems' base with diameters of 1 1/2 inches or less. On walls, they may even be loosely scattered to dry.

3. Barks: Peel the exterior bark off if necessary. Here it is named flipping.

4. Roots: Stretch them out or circle. Rinsing can usually not remove soil particles. A pressure hose is sometimes necessary, as well as hand brushing, especially with clay. Cut lengthwise for long, heavy roots without aromatic properties.5. Both plant elements, when delicate, are dry. In the lower portion, pinch the hanging trees. Break a broad specimen root in half to see if the heart is dry.

1.6Defensive Tips-Using and misusing herbs

The German-Swiss physicist & alchemist Paracelsus and the herbalist, physician, and astrologer Nicholas Culpepper developed positions in botanical plant pharmacy, mathematics, alchemy, and astrology in the 16th and 17th centuries. While in today's legitimized occupations, the naturopathic elements of botany and mathematics have been added, astrology and alchemy appear to others merely superstition. But to build a comprehensive method of studying, understanding, and utilizing plant medicine in conflicting ways, this mixture of studies is required. Scientific science has allowed us today to investigate herbs, their properties, and how they act as natural remedies as they are used. Herbal treatments have been checked and validated time and again in order to produce the same results. Several herbs have been extensively researched, and there is no doubt that they are powerful and healthy and have calming properties. Herbal science and regulation are hot topics, and I'm not big on these topics in my job, truth be told. Therefore, the study will serve to further the use of plant medicines and to educate and raise knowledge of herbs' medicinal properties. I deal for the general public, and my herb shop is visited every day by a wide variety of individuals, from many who know little about herbs to professionally qualified herbalists. Every entity needs scientific knowledge of how plants function within the body, and they are suspicious of natural therapies without this.

Perhaps further study will open doors for those who, by traditional approaches, are less capable of learning about herbs. It is vital to bear in mind that not all experiments are precise. Nonetheless, search for details on every analysis you read. Why has the examination taken? On one part of the plant or the whole item, was the appraisal done? Will the researcher make or sell a product appropriate to the examination that is advertised? This understanding will offer useful advice about whether, depending on the objectives, the study is factual or subjective. If you wish to support your herbal study interests, we suggest the American Botanical Council (abc.herbalgram.org) & the work of its chairman, the herbalist Mark Blumenthal.

1.7The Ultimate Thread

Use these American Indian herbal remedies to your benefit. Now that the secrets of these therapeutic herbs in Native America have been unlocked, individuals will start using them to boost their immunity, improve their cognitive ability, and treat several health issues.

As first-line therapy, most people prefer plants as a drug instead of drugs. Since these herbal treatments offer a healthy and convenient way to improve well-being, this makes common sense. Instead, if you pick supplements to avoid the short and long-term adverse effects correlated with prescribed medications, then do you select drugs?

Sacred Native Americans and There Herbal Remedies

The indigenous tribes of America have relied on the medicinal benefits of herbs for centuries. Now it's time to take a closer look at Native America's herbal medicines and the important nutritional benefits they can bring. What you may not realize is that these natural supplements are divine & highly compensated ownership, largely because of their natural healing ability. The American Indians kept knowledge regarding the usage & advantages of the plants so close to their bosom that sharing was forbidden, except among the different tribes.

You will assess the potential health benefits of the following medicinal herbs from Native America in this chapter:

1. Echinacea: the modern cold, immunity, skin disorders

2. Black Cohosh: hot sweats, rheumatism, nausea, arthritis, fever (menopause)

3. Saw Palmetto: prostate gland and urinary tract, libido, hair loss

4. Yarrow: injuries & burns, respiratory system diseases, skin disorders, insomnia, fear.

5. American ginseng: protection, the efficiency of memory, tension, cancer

6. Club of the Devil: body and bone discomfort, skin abnormalities, cancer

7. Nettle: digestion, swelling, and nausea, asthma, high blood pressure

Different indigenous groups have used these seven medicinal plants for centuries, and a few of them form the base of many modern medicines & remedies. A safe way to improve immunity and alleviate a list of diseases such as headache, cough, discomfort, rashes, fever, and nausea has been given by these herbs.

Historians claim that awareness of herbal medicine is culturally preserved because it includes natural secrets of healing for common illnesses that doctors treat with pharmaceuticals today. Invariably, the secrets of these spiritual cures were eventually uncovered, and scientists started to research these plants to thoroughly understand their uses & healing properties. When you hear about these fascinating herbs, you'll definitely want to try out some of them. Another choice is to track the tribes and pick herbs from the wild in their footsteps.

However, this needs certain specialized expertise to guarantee the pickup of the correct farm. Users ought to know about handling the herbs prior to using them. And, of course, the unique herb has to be accessible near where you reside. A more effective way of consuming these medicinal plants is to purchase ready-made teas & supplements. To make it simpler, we have mentioned the best possible products for each plant in this chapter here.

There are a number of items to bear in mind until you begin using some of the herbs. Any herbal remedies can interact with prescription and over-the-counter (OTC) drugs, as well as other herbal items. If you are on medication or have chronic illnesses, before taking any herbal supplements, you can still speak to your doctor or a trained health care provider, while the usage of these plants is generally deemed healthy.

2.1Echinacea

Echinacea purpurea, also called the American coneflower, is another American Indian meditative herb worth noting. There are nine plant types utilized by the Great Plains region's tribal communities.

Two species that are widespread are Echinacea purpurea & Echinacea Angustifolia. This herb is commonly used today as well, and its usefulness has been verified by many reports. The fruits, leaves, and roots of this potent plant have wide-ranging medicinal advantages owing to its anti-inflammatory & anti-viral effects.

Native Americans, like the Kiowa & Cheyenne, have historically used Echinacea to treat cold symptoms such as coughs and sore throats. They munched the roots or used dried roots to produce a tea that has anti-viral properties. They have also used coneflower as a natural treatment for discomfort, high blood pressure, and inflammation.

A great deal of study has been conducted on Echinacea in order to assess its medicinal efficacy and usefulness in the treatment of symptoms of common cold & upper respiratory tract infections. This herb will help avoid and cure upper respiratory infections such as colds, based on a study of 16 trials.

There is a lot of other evidence confirming the effectiveness of Echinacea as an influenza drug. By consuming Echinacea at the onset of the cold, the frequency of symptoms may be substantially decreased. It may also lower the likelihood of recurring respiratory infections and their related complications.

Currently, herbalists, naturopathic doctors, and customers utilize Echinacea as a nutritional supplement & alternative solution to cure and avoid common cold symptoms. The herb's amazing healing properties tend to enhance the immune system's work and boost the body's capacity to successfully fight infection. One research shows that the plant may be a supplement for battling cancer because of the strong phytochemicals it contains.

In addition to using this herb as an extract or tea to treat cuts, rashes, & other skin disorders, Echinacea formulations can be used topically (applied to the skin).

Some of the finest Echinacea items available are in the market are as follows:

Organic Echinacea + Traditional Medicinal Tea: To improve the immune system and to stop getting ill, you will heartily suggest this flavorful tea. There are also small quantities of lemongrass and spearmint in it.

Nature's Abundance Echinacea Capsules: Utilizing these inexpensive and affordable capsules is the easiest way to explore Echinacea's health benefits.

Horbaach Echinacea Liquid Extract: A perfect way to get a shot of this immune-boosting herb is to combine few drops of liquid extract with a cup of water or juice.

2.2Black Cohosh

The Black Cohosh, Actaea racemosa, comes from eastern North America and is a flowering herb. It is a member of the buttercup family (Ranunculaceae) and goes by other names such as snakeroot, rattle root, bugbane, and squaw base.Native Americans admire this herb because of its capacity to relieve disorders such as fever, rheumatism, discomfort, arthritis, and rattlesnake bite. Traditionally, it has been used for gynecological disorders, as the word "squaw root" suggests. It may be used to improve menstrual discharge with premenopausal, multiple menstrual, and menopausal symptoms.There is empirical research in support of the therapeutic assertions of black cohosh. It is especially useful in managing hot flashes that may last for years before (perimenopause) and after the time of menopause. They can cause severe depression and are responsible for insomnia, anxiety, and diminished quality of life of many women.

In the prevention of hot flashes, a 2018 report checked the potency of black cohosh and indicated that the herb is very effective in managing this symptom. The research was done on 80 postmenopausal women who had been offered the herb for eight weeks. The researchers determined that black cohosh decreased the intensity of hot flashes and effectively increased the life dominance of the members.

It may also help control the development of estrogen in women because black cohosh influences female hormones. The findings of one study acknowledge that the usage of this herb is a possible prevention step against breast cancer initiation & progression.

This herb was also used to cause labor by traditional herbal physicians. It is also not advised for pregnant people, since it can end up triggering labor to begin accidentally. In capsules, extracts, tinctures, herbal teas, and several other kinds, it is possible to use black cohosh as a dried root.

Some of the preferred items made of black cohosh are as follows:

This high-quality herbal tea has a gentle earthy taste and consists of 100 percent raw black cohosh root. Organic Black Cohosh Tea (Buddha Teas):

Nature's Way Black Cohosh Root Capsules: If you like consuming this herb in a tablet, ordering these GMO & gluten-free capsules is suggested.

2.3The Palmetto Saw

A type of tree (palm) that grows in the southeast of the United States is Serenoa repens. Historically, North

American Indians have used this plant's berries for intestinal pain, inflammation, digestion, and a variety of urinary tract diseases in persons. Some of them thought that the berries increased male levels of testosterone, sperm production, and libido.

In 92 older Chinese males with urinary tract infection associated with BPH (benign prostate hyperplasia) or noncancerous enlarged prostate, a clinical trial was performed. They were given soft gel (Prostataplex) palmetto capsules for 12 weeks. The results of the trials suggest that palmetto may have little effect on the recovery of urinary tract symptoms.

There is also evidence that this herbal treatment may play a role in preventing prostate cancer by delaying the development of a hormone called dihydrotestosterone (DHT) into a hormone (powerful androgen).

As per a 2009 study, saw palmetto can also support males and females suffering alopecia (hair loss). After 3 months of utilizing shampoo and lotion containing Serenoa repens (SR) extract, the test participants reported an increase in hair density.

Herbal items extracted from dried berries & tablets manufactured from saw palmetto extract are also on the market. They are commonly used in males to monitor hormones, encourage prostate protection, and decrease hair loss.

Organic Saw Palmetto tea is suggested to make a smooth & tasty drink with a healthy, natural remedy as the ideal choice (Buddha Teas). Try saw-palmetto capsules if you want an alternative.

2.4 The Yarrow

Yarrow, Achillea millefolium, is one of the most widespread medicinal plants worldwide and is an aromatic flowering herb. The plant, a.k.a., woundwort of a soldier, got its name from the tale used for its wounds by the Greek hero, Achilles.

The flowers, leaves, and stems of this plant were collected by the aboriginal North American people and used them primarily to treat wounds, injuries, respiratory illnesses, reduce excessive bleeding, skin limitations, irritation, and insomnia.

The Yarrow of the Rosa

Yarrow has many other positive benefits, including the effects of metabolism and sedation on well-being. To cure a disturbed stomach & other gastrointestinal issues, Indians combined fresh yarrow juice with water to start with. The tribes often used the plant's leaves to create a liquid that they used as an astringent.

Thanks to its antioxidant and anti-inflammatory effects, Yarrow is praised for its wound & skin-healing ability. An analysis performed by Ethnopharmacology globally examined the topical application of the anti-inflammatory ability of the yarrow oil extract and concluded that it had good anti-inflammatory properties. It can help to cure multiple skin conditions owing to Yarrow's protective impact on the skin's pH & its anti-inflammatory agents.

This plant, obtained from the findings of various trials, can also be a potential herbal alternative for high blood pressure & anxiety. Researchers evaluated yarrow extract's anxiolytic-like properties and noticed that it would have anti-anxiety effects close to those found in diazepam, a medication commonly used to alleviate anxiety.

Yarrow tea has a bitter smell, so if you don't mind, go ahead and get some Buddha Tea Organic Yarrow Tea. This 100% organic yarrow oil is accessible and it is possible to play with it.

2.5 America Ginseng

Panax quinquefolius (American ginseng) is treasured as one of the most excellent American Indian herbal treatments and is one of the top five most popular medicines of the Seneca tribe. The herb is also a member of the Araliaceous plant family and is distinct from Siberian ginseng, also known as Panax ginseng, also known as Eleuthero coccus senticosus & Asian/Korean ginseng.

The American Ginseng Root

American ginseng was a natural remedy for the tribal people who used it for millennia as a cure for swelling, fever, erectile dysfunction, tension and improving the sex desire of males and females.

Unlike Asian ginseng and all its "warming" properties, Conventional Chinese Medicine categorizes American ginseng as a "cooling" or soothing tonic that can be used to support stress-related patients.

Including good anti-cancer effects, this plant has broad-based benefits. American research into the root of ginseng suggests that it has the potential to combat cancer, especially colorectal cancer. In other research, American ginseng has been shown to have anti-diabetic, anti-viral, and anti-inflammatory health benefits. There is proof that it will reduce blood sugar levels and decrease the incidence of cold and flu symptoms in people with type 2 diabetes.

American ginseng is also able to improve immune cell efficiency to protect the body against many disorders and infections. A 2017 study indicates that using ginseng can offer you a higher chance of a disease-free life.

Finally, the analysis found that it can be used to improve emotional energy and cognitive efficiency levels. As such, it is used by scientists as a possible herbal cure for situations that trigger diminished cognitive capacity, such as Alzheimer's disease.

Such remarkable American ginseng products:

American Ginseng Tea from Baumann: This tea has a lovely and slightly sweet flavor and is produced from American ginseng.

NOW Supplements American Ginseng Capsules: With these inexpensive and excellent capsules, get an appropriate dose of ginseng.

American Ginseng Tincture: If users desire to use ginseng in a form of liquid that is absorbed rapidly, this is the better choice.

2.6The Devil's Club

In western North America, the wild herb Devil's club (Oplopanax horridus), also called the Devil's walking stick, is a sacred native shape. The root was munched, the bark fermented, or a potion was prepared and used for a multitude of things, such as moral defense, to produce a medicinal drink.

Rewards from Devil's Club

The inner bark & seeds of the Devil's club are used medicinally for colds, TB, allergies, stomach disorders, skin infections, pain & inflammation of arthritis. This is not shocking after observing that the herb has anti-viral, anti-fungal, anti-bacterial, & anti-mycobacterial effects, given phytochemical research. The most detailed study on the Devil's club was conducted to determine the potential to combat cancer. There have been suggestions that certain cancer cells may inhibit the growth of the root bark extract.

To alleviate discomfort and frustration, you can use the Club Salve of the Snowy Summit Devil and add it to achy muscles and joints. It is also beneficial with rashes, minor burns and insect bites to be treated. Herb Pharm Devil's Club Liquid Extract is another outstanding product manufactured from the root bark of wildcrafted Oplopanax horridus in the Pacific Northwest.

2.7Nettle

Nettle is another herb that has undoubtedly earned its spot in our Native American herbal remedies collection.

Urtica dioica (Stinging nettle) belongs to the Urticaceae family and there is a long history of medicinal usage by American Indians.

It appears to be an ordinary herb, however, due to its antioxidant and anti-inflammatory effects, as well as a vast variety of phytochemicals contained in different areas of the plant, it has an excessive healing ability.

Ventajas with Nettle

Historically, Urtica dioica has been used to relieve skin disorders such as psoriasis and eczema. Men also have nettle rubbed on their bodies ceremonially to protect them when hunting, since it produces a stinging feeling.

The Cherokee used the root for a troubled stomach, while it was used for colds, coughs, swelling, asthma, and rheumatism by other tribes. In order to prevent hemorrhaging, native herbal doctors also gave nettle to pregnant women, although breastfeeding mothers used it to improve milk production.

Recent laboratory experiments have shown that the stinging nettle is a plant capable of treating asthma, disease, inflammation of the urinary tract, prostate enlargement that is not cancerous, and high blood pressure. It may be used to tackle seasonal conditions as well. One study verified this plant's antihypertensive function and recommended it as a potential medication for high blood pressure treatment.

Recommended Nettle Products:

Organic Nettle Leaf Tea (Buddha Teas): Try this nettle leaf tea with a smooth taste and experience the inherent potential for healing.

Real Herbs Stinging Nettle Root Extract Capsules: For enhancing urinary tract & prostate well-being, this incredibly potent, US-made medication is excellent.

Nature's Response Liquid Nettles Extract: A perfect choice if you want to use an easy-to-digest nettle leaf meal.

Native Americans Widely Used Medicinal Plants

Native Americans are acclaimed for their medicinal plant knowledge. Since animals eat these plants when they are wounded, it is rumored that they first started to use plants and herbs for healing. In order to protect these plants from over-harvesting, the medicine men used to collect every third plant they encountered. Native Americans have a philosophical viewpoint on existence, and in order to be good, a person will have to have a philosophy of purpose and follow a rational, harmonious, and balanced path in life. They thought that such disorders were life lessons to be learned by the person & that they could not interfere. Several modern treatments & medications are based on the Native American understanding of the many plants and herbs they have used for centuries.

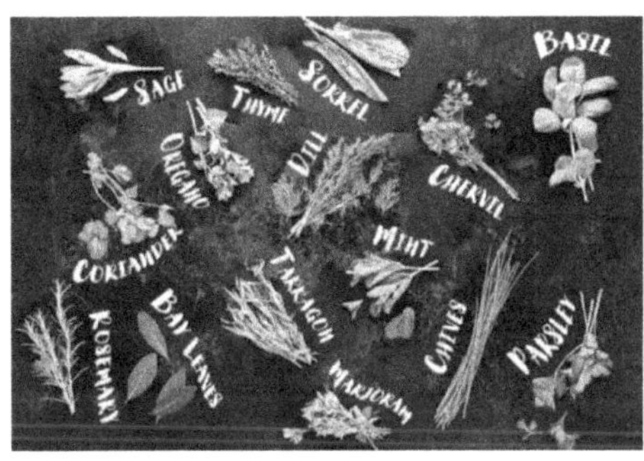

Here are the most mobile plants used by Native Americans during their everyday lives:

3.1 The Blackberries

The Cherokee used this herb to ease a troubled stomach. They used blackberry to cure diarrhea and soothe sore tissues & joints (tea). Combined with honey or maple syrup, blackberry root can create an all-natural cough remedy to treat sore throats. To soothe gum infections, they have used the leaves to suck (bleeding). Sometimes, to strengthen the whole immune system, this plant is perfect.

3.2Sumac

In various herbal remedies, this plant may be used, but this is one of the few plants used to remedy eye problems by healers. A sumac decoction was used as a gargle to cure sore throats or taken as a diarrhea remedy. The leaves and berries were blended into tea or made into a potion to soothe poison ivy in order to alleviate fever.

3.3The Mint

The Cherokee used to create a mint tea to pacify digestion symptoms and help an irritated stomach. A salve was also made from its leaves to treat sore skin and rashes.

3.4Rosemary

Native American tribes found this herb to be sacred. They used it mostly as an analgesic for relieving sore muscles. This herb improves concentration, relieves muscle pain and spasms, and stimulates the circulatory & nervous systems. Therefore, the immune reaction is reinforced, and indigestion is treated.

3.5The Bark of Black Gum

The Cherokee also used to produce light tea from twigs & black gum bark to ease chest pains.

3.6Clover of the Red

This herb has also been used by healers to cure asthma & respiratory issues. The new studies have shown that red clover helps prevent heart risk by increasing breathing and reducing cholesterol.

3.7Greenbriar

To purify blood or to relieve joint pain, this root tea has been used. A salve combined with hog lard from leaves and bark was generated by some healers, which was applied to mild sores, scalds, & burns.

3.8Cattail

This is one of the most common medicinal plants used by indigenous people for food and also as defensive medicine. It helps to recover from illness, as it is a food that is easily digestible. Because it can be used in numerous dishes, it is named the swamp supermarket.

3.9Sage

Sage is commonly used as a seasoning, but it was a sacred plant for many indigenous populations as it was thought to have strong purifying energies & to cleanse the body of toxic energy. To tackle medical conditions such as abdominal cramps, spasms, fractures, wounds, colds, and influenza, it has been used as a remedy.

3.10Hummingbird Blossom

The American Indians used this herb, also known as the buck brush, in order to treat mouth and throat issues, as well as cysts, fibroid tumors, & inflammation. It may be turned into a potion to help in treating wounds, sores, & injuries. A diuretic that increases kidney function may be developed using the roots of such an herb. The early colonists used this unusual plant as a substitute for black tea. The new studies have also shown that The Buck Brush is helpful in controlling the lymph stream's elevated blood pressure & blockages.

3.11The Elm Slippery

The Native Americans made bowstrings, yarn, fabric, and rope using the inner bark. Tea was developed to soothe toothaches, nasal irritations, skin issues, intestinal pain, sore throats, and even leaf and bark spider bites.

3.12The Rose of the Wild

This herb was used as a preventive and a remedy for mild common cold by Native Americans. For the bladder & kidneys, the tea stimulates and is a mild diuretic. For a sore throat, a petal injection was used.

3.13Ginger of the Wild

To treat earaches & ear infections, this herb is used by healers. They also found a gentle tea for the rootstock to stimulate the digestive system & reduce bloating and it also aids in bronchial diseases and exhaustion.

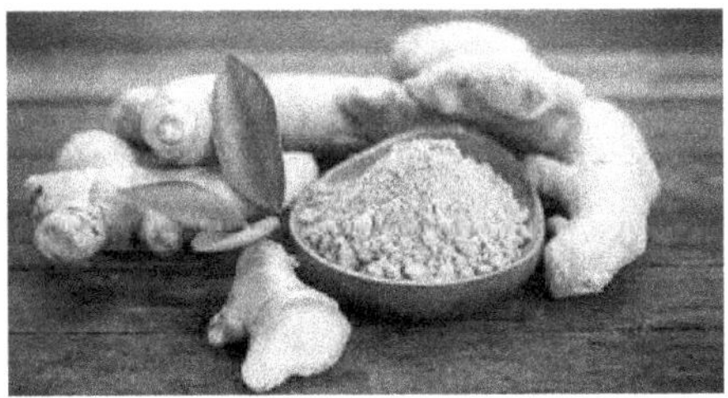

3.14Lavender

This herb has been used by healers as a medication for fatigue, anxiety, tension, headaches, and exhaustion. In the essential oil, antiseptic & anti-inflammatory properties are found. Infusions can be used to soothe insect bites and burns.

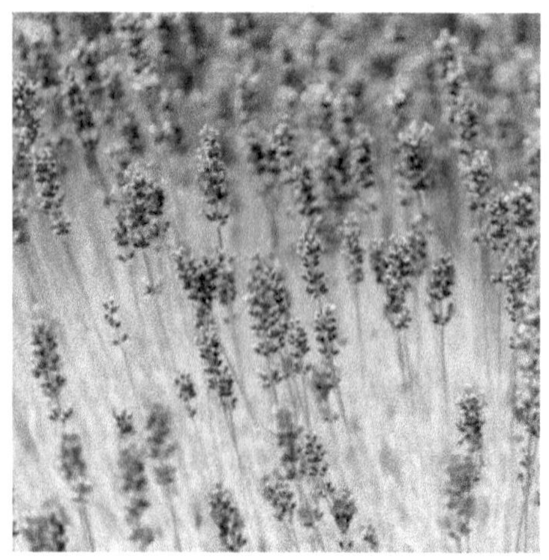

3.15Honeysuckle

Native Americans used this plant as a natural medicine to treat asthma, but it has many medical applications, including hepatitis, rheumatoid arthritis, and mumps. It helps in upper respiratory tract infections, such as pneumonia, as well.

3.16Cactus of the Prickly Pear

This plant is used both as a diet and as a medicine. Native Americans produced a poultice from developed sheets as an antiseptic & for treating burns, boils, and wounds. Tea was developed to treat the infections of urine and to improve the immune system. The study further shows that cholesterol can be decreased and heart failure and diet-related diabetes can be avoided.

3.17Mullein

It was a tobacco-like plant and was mainly used for the treatment of respiratory disorders. Native Americans made concoctions from the roots in order to alleviate swelling in the joints, paws, or feet.

3.18Ashwagandha

This plant was important for healers because of its various unusual medicinal uses. It tackles bone weakness, muscle wasting, and stiffness, missing teeth, loss of recollection, & rheumatism. And as a sedative, it can be used. It also has an ultimate rejuvenating effect on the body if it improves stamina. Using the leaves and root bark as an antibiotic is often crucial. When made into a poultice, it helps to reduce swelling and controls pain. Caution is advised when utilizing this plant as it is toxic.

3.19Uva Ursi

It is also known as Bearberry & Bear grape, due to the affection of the bear for this plant's fruits. Native Americans used this herb mainly to treat bladder & urinary tract diseases.

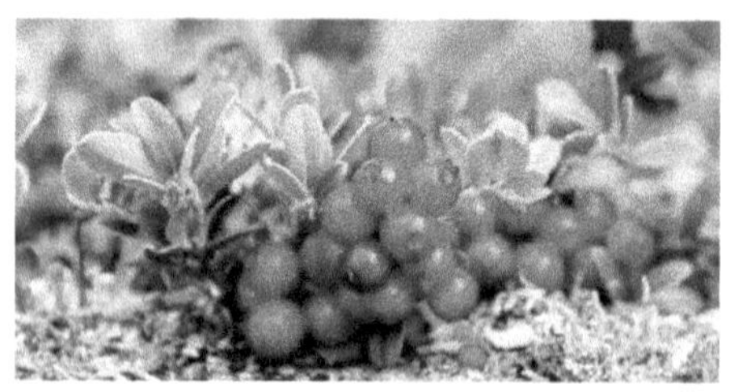

3.20Claw of the Devil

It was used by the American Indians to treat various ailments, from treating fever to calming skin conditions, enhancing metabolism, and controlling arthritis, whereas a toxic plant may be suggested by the name. While a concoction made from the plant's roots prevents stiffness and helps with sores, joint disease, gout, back pain, headache, and arthritis, the effects of diabetes may be reduced through tea. Notice that although medical treatment is not accessible, knowledge is the only doctor that will save you.

3.21The Origin of Licorice

This root is commonly used for flavoring candies, foods, and beverages. But it has also been used by healers to treat stomach disorders, bronchitis, food poisoning, and chronic fatigue.

3.22Salix (Willow)

Both the Greeks and American Indians valued Willow bark as pain relief and among the first therapeutic substances to be collected from plants in 1852 was the active ingredient of the herb, salicin. It proved to be a successful pain reliever, yet weakened the stomach sufficiently to form a drug that is now manufactured as aspirin, which is identical and safer.

3.23Rosy Periwinkle (Catharanthus Roseus)

Both parts of the plant are venomous. In Rosy periwinkle, there are many compounds of therapeutic potential, two of which, vincristine & vinblastine, are important drugs in the treatment of leukemia and certain other cancers.

3.24Yew (Taxus Baccata)

The Pacific yew from North America (Northwest) was used by Native Americans to treat skin cancer. Clinical study has shown that Taxol, a medicine that has become an effective treatment for cancer of the breast, ovary & cervix, is included. Fortunately, English yews were found to have a certain compound that could be turned into Taxol in their leaves, and pharmaceutical companies are collecting yew hedge clippings for this purpose.

3.25Chamomile (The Flower)

In the United States, chamomile is widely used for anxiety & relaxation as an anxiolytic & sedative, considered by few to be a cure-all. In Europe, it is used for wound healing and to minimize swelling and inflammation. Few trials have investigated how well it operates for any disease. Chamomile is used or used as a compress as tea. It is considered safe by the FDA. Sleepiness triggered by drugs or other herbs or supplements can increase. Chamomile may interfere with the way the body uses other medications, allowing the amount of medication to be too big in certain persons. Speak, as for any medicinal plant, with the healthcare provider before taking it.

3.26Garlic (Root Cloves)

For cholesterol levels & control of blood pressure, garlic is used. It has antimicrobial effects. Reports from minor, short-term, & badly defined trials suggest that slight decreases may be induced by total & LDL cholesterol. The German research results on garlic's cholesterol-lowering influence have been distorted, however, with a positive result, the FDA says. The possible role of garlic in cancer prevention is currently being studied by researchers. The FDA considers garlic to be safe. It should not be mixed with warfarin, since large amounts of garlic can induce clotting. Big doses must not be administered until oral surgery or surgery for the same reason.

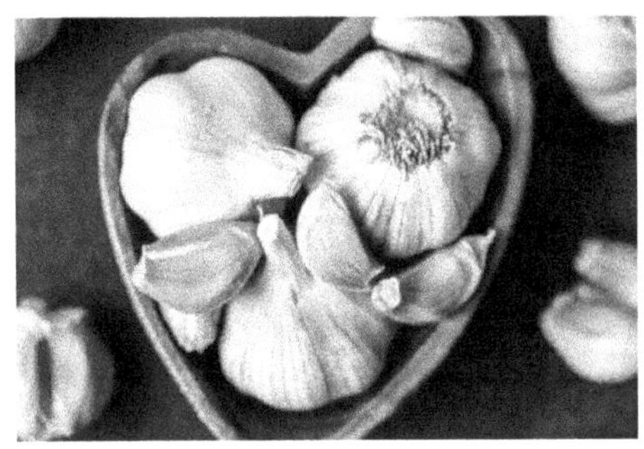

3.27Feverfew (The Leaf)

Historically, Feverfew has been used as a cure for fever. In order to treat arthritis and alleviate migraines, it is still commonly used. Any evidence has indicated that migraines can be avoided with any feverfew preparedness. Among the adverse effects are oral ulcers & abdominal pain. People who suddenly avoid taking feverfew for migraines can have their headaches returned. It cannot be used with nonsteroidal anti-inflammatory drugs since these drugs can impact how well feverfew performs. In tandem with warfarin and other anticoagulant drugs, it cannot be used.

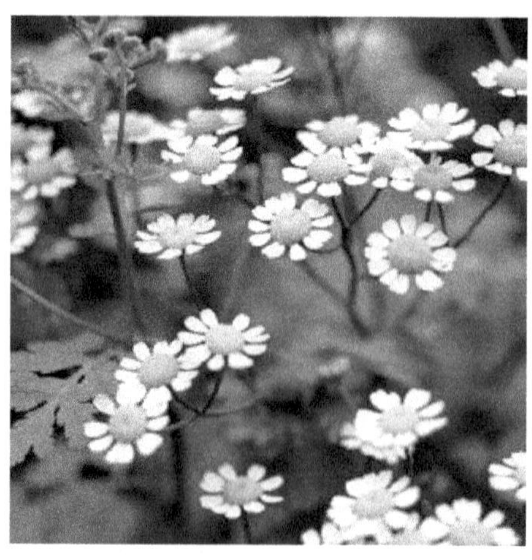

3.28The Ginger (The Root)

Ginger is used to minimizing pain & motion sickness. The study indicates that ginger could decrease pain caused by pregnancy and chemotherapy. Surgery and motion-induced nausea are implicated in these areas under review. Gas, bloating, heartburn, and nausea are among the side effects identified.

3.29Goldenseal (Rhizome, Racine)

Goldenseal is used in the treatment of eye and skin diarrhea & itching. It is used in the context of an antiseptic. It is also an unproven treatment for colds. In Goldenseal, berberine, an herbal alkaloid with a long history of medicinal use in both Ayurvedic and Chinese medicine, is contained. The efficacy of Goldenseal for diarrhea has been proven by research. But it's not allowed because it could be unsafe in broad quantities.

Skin, mouth, stomach, & gastric pain may be enticing. It is not recommended, even because of the plant's endangered species status.

2.30Ginseng (The Root)

As a tonic & aphrodisiac, ginseng is used as a cure-all as well. The analysis remains uncertain regarding how well it does, mainly owing to the difficulty in defining "vitality" and "quality of life." The accuracy of sold ginseng varies greatly. Side effects include elevated blood pressure & tachycardia. The FDA finds it safe, but it is difficult to use heparin, warfarin, nonsteroidal anti-inflammatory drugs, estrogens, corticosteroids, or digoxin for it. People with diabetes shouldn't use Ginseng.

2.31The Thistle of Milk (The Fruit)

Milk thistle is used to cure complications with the liver and high cholesterol and to decrease the development of cancer cells. It emerged in the region of the Mediterranean. It has been used for many different diseases, especially liver problems, for the past few thousand years. There are some promising data, but the results of the study are vague.

2.32Valeriano (The Root)

For sleeplessness treatment and anxiety relief, Valerian is included. Research suggests that valerian can be a helpful sleep aid, but there have been no well-designed research to support the claims. Valerian is used as a flavoring for root beer as well as other foods in the United States. Speak, as for any medicinal plant, with the medical professional before taking it.

2.33The Wort of Saint John (Flower, Leaf)

Saint John's Wort is deemed an antidepressant. The latest studies have not shown that depression has more than a tiny effect. Further testing is needed to determine the right dose. A side effect is an exposure to light, but this is often found in people consuming large doses of the medication.

St. John's Wort can cause a dangerous association with other commonly used drugs. Please contact the healthcare practitioner prior to eating this plant.

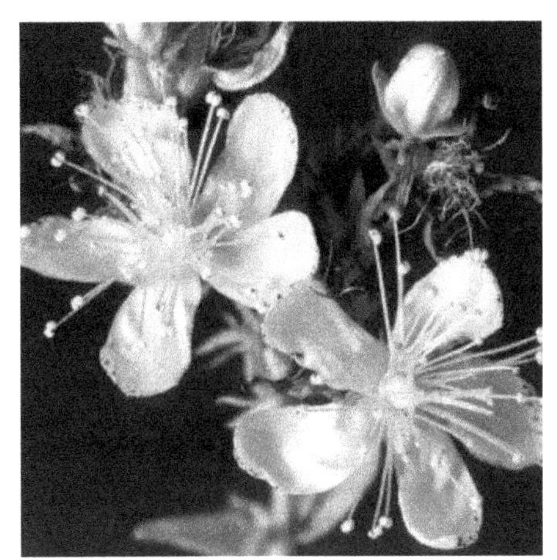

Unadventurous Illness and Natural Medications

This chapter addresses many of the most common diseases and remedies that Native Americans find for us. Everything about it is analyzed in detail.

4.1The Acne

Acne develops when microbes obstruct or corrupt pores. In the United States, acne is the most prevalent skin disease, affecting nearly 80% of people in their lives.

To help control oil levels in the skin, relieve inflammation, destroy bacteria, and avoid potential acne breakouts, people can use particular home remedies.

Popular Acne Remedies

For some of the more common acne remedies, the use of herbal medicinal extracts, some of which have been used by traditional medicine practitioners for hundreds of years, is needed.

Below, we address the safest home remedies for acne, what the evidence suggests, and the behavioral improvements that could improve.

1. Oil of Tea Tree

Tea tree oil is a natural anti-inflammatory and antibacterial agent, meaning that it is possible to destroy P. acnes, the bacteria that cause acne. The anti-inflammatory effects of tea tree oil indicate that it can also reduce pimple redness and inflammation.

The established evidence for tea tree oil & acne was looked at in a 2015 study report. The researchers noticed that tea tree oil products can reduce acne sores in people with mild to severe acne.

When someone should use oil from a tea tree

In creams, gels, and essential oils, individuals might add tea tree oil to their acne. They often first dilute them in a carrier liquid when essential oils are used by humans.

2. Oil derived from Jojoba

Jojoba oil is the natural, waxy material of jojoba gained from the (shrub) plants. The waxy constituents in the oil of jojoba can help regenerate the skin that is damaged, which means that, like acne lesions, it can also help enhance wound healing.

Any of the compounds of jojoba oil can help alleviate skin irritation, ensuring that redness & swelling around the pimples, whiteheads, and other irritating lesions can be minimized.

Researchers gave 133 individuals clay face masks that included jojoba oil in a 2012 report. Individuals reported a 54 percent improvement in their acne following six weeks of wearing the masks two to three days a week.

How to Make Use of Jojoba Oil

Try to blend jojoba essential oil with clay face mask cream or gel and add it to the acne. Otherwise, on a cotton pad, put a few drops of jojoba oil and gently massage it into acne sores.

3. Aloe of Vera

Aloe Vera is an effective anti-inflammatory and antibacterial medication that ensures that it is possible to decrease the presence of acne & avoid acne breakouts.

An excellent moisturizer containing watercolors is Aloe Vera since it is particularly desirable for people who may have their skin dry from a range of other products that are anti-acne.

In a 2014 study, researchers supplied individuals with moderate to mild aloe Vera acne gel & tretinoin cream to use for eight weeks with a popular O.T.C. acne treatment. In comparison to persons who used only tretinoin gel, the researchers showed a significant improvement in both inflammatory and non-inflammatory acne.

Aloe Vera gel Usage

Aim to disinfect the acne sores & then add at least ten percent of the Aloe Vera content to a thin coat of cream or gel.

4. Honey

For thousands of years, honey has been used to cure skin conditions, such as acne. It includes several antioxidants that can help clear clogged pores from waste and debris. Owing to its antibacterial & wound-healing abilities, physicians use honey in dressings.

Honey Utilization

Massage a touch of honey onto the pimples with a clean finger/cotton pad. Or else, apply the face or body mask with honey.

5. Garlic

Sometimes, garlic is used by traditional medicine practitioners to cure illnesses and improve the body's ability to resist germs and diseases.N Garlic develops organosulfur compounds that have anti-inflammatory and antibacterial properties that are normal. Organosulfur compounds, which enable the body to avoid infections, may also strengthen the immune system.

Using cloves

People should incorporate enough garlic into their diet to combat the inflammation & infections induced by acne. Some people chew whole cloves of garlic, sprinkle them on toast, or turn them into a fiery drink.

Customers can also obtain garlic powder or tablets from most shops and natural health shops.

6. Leaf Tea Around

Green tea includes a category of polyphenol antioxidants named catechism in substantial quantities. There are so many sebum oils and natural body oils in the pores of certain people with acne, just not enough antioxidants.

Antioxidants enable the body to break down compounds that can affect healthy cells from chemicals & waste products. Any of the residues & waste accumulated in exposed acne sores may be removed by green tea.

There are also compounds in green tea which can help:

- Lower the development of sebum in the skin
- P. acne minimized

- Inflammation removal
- Make use of green tea

Green tea can benefit when people drink it or use green tea on their faces, but researchers claim there is no current evidence.

However, after eight weeks of utilizing polyphenol green tea extract, one study found a 79 to 89 percent drop in whiteheads and blackheads.

7. The Echinacea

Compounds, such as P. acnes, also known as purple coneflower, can be present in Echinacea purpurea, which helps eradicate bacteria and viruses.

Many people claim that Echinacea, including colds and flu, can strengthen the immune system and reduce inflammation, and therefore use it to deter or prevent diseases.

How to Enable Echinacea to be used

People should add Echinacea-containing creams to places where they have acne spots or where they have supplements of Echinacea.

8. Rosemary

Rosemary extract includes chemicals and substances that have antibacterial, antioxidant, and anti-inflammatory properties or have Rosmarinus officinalis.The impact of rosemary extract on acne has been studied in a few studies; however, a 2013 report on mice models and human cells showed that rosemary extract can decrease inflammation from the P. acnes bacteria that cause acne.

9. Venom Fermented Bee

It has been shown that purified bee venom contains antibacterial properties. Researchers disclosed in a 2013 analysis that purified bee venom might really kill P. acne bacteria. Changes in the number of acne lesions are seen in people that have used products containing derived bee venom for two weeks. In a 2016 report, people who for six weeks applied a gel containing bee venom (purified) to their face saw a drop in acne lesions that were mild to moderate. While further testing is needed, distilled bee venom may be a helpful potential component of acne medicine.

10. Oil for Cocos

Coconut oil produces anti-inflammatory & antibacterial agents, much as other natural remedies.

These characteristics indicate that coconut oil may destroy bacteria that cause acne and minimize pimple redness & swelling. The treatment of open acne sores can also be accelerated by coconut oil.

How to Use Coconut Oil Optimized?

Try rubbing the acne region directly with pure, virgin coconut oil.

Lifestyle changes for acne

Relevant lifestyle improvements, along with home remedies, may have a significant effect on maintaining the body safe, rendering the skin a lesser amount of oily, & decreasing acne flare-ups.

11. Don't touch pimples

This may be really attractive, but it can irritate the skin by touching acne sores, making the pimple deeper, and expanding pimples to other places.

More bacteria may also be injected into the lesion by squeezing, grinding, splitting, or bursting acne sores, producing more infections.

Bacteria & debris may be forced deeper into the skin by squeezing a pimple such that the pimple can come back worse than ever.

12. Using skincare that is oil-free

Pores may be blocked by oil-based or greasy fabrics, raising the possibility of clogging and causing acne sores.

Look for skincare items & cosmetics marketed as 'oil-free' or 'non-comedogenic,' which contain ingredients that allow pores to breathe.

13. To remain hydrated

It is highly necessary to remain hydrated as it allows acne sores to recover more easily and reduces the potential chance of outbreaks.

When the skin is dry, which results in pimples, it may easily become uncomfortable or injured. When sores recover, getting hydrated often means the fresh skin cells grow properly.

There is no regular everyday water consumption dosage and the individual's water requirements are different based on age, how healthy they are, weather, and any medical conditions.

Many health officials estimate that six to eight-ounce glasses of liquid are drunk regularly.

14. Relief from pressures

As a potential cause of acne flare-ups, tension is recognized by the American Academy of Dermatology.

Stress causes the hormone androgen concentrations to climb. Androgen reduces the risk of acne by enhancing hair follicles & oil glands in the pores.

Tips on stress-management include:

- Speak to parents, peers, a counselor, or other helpful people
- Getting a daily, nutritious meal and not missing meals
- Acquiring adequate sleep
- Normal exercise
- The practice of yoga, profound healing, contemplation, or consciousness
- Limiting intake of alcohol and caffeine
- Valid acne-related facilities

There are several alternatives for acne medical care, all of which are extremely effective, but they do have some adverse results and may not be suitable for everybody.

People should speak to a doctor about whether pharmaceutical or medicinal creams, especially if natural treatments have not succeeded, are correct for them to use.

The following active ingredients are used in conventional O.T.C. treatments against mild-moderate acne sores:

- Salicylic Acid
- Hydrogen peroxide
- Hydroxyl alpha-acids

Individuals should choose from a large range of home remedies in order to cure their acne. Not all techniques, though, would succeed on anyone or under some situations.

To figure out which methods function for them, people will choose to use trial and error. Plant products or essential oils are not monitored by the U.S.F.D.A. (Food and Drug Administration).

It is not statistically proven that any natural acne treatments are successful, though some people can find them helpful.

4.2Allergies

The effects may be mitigated by over-the-counter medications, while certain alternative remedies can also function. Here is a couple to start seeking.

Herb Supplements

In the shape of a pad, a fall, or tea, you can get this.

It is claimed that in your pantry you can also have one verified allergy tracker: "Green tea is a pure antihistamine that is potent enough to potentially help with allergy skin checking." Drink two cups a day to help alleviate congestion, around two weeks before the allergy season begins.

The plant, called butterbur, will resist allergies and over-the-counter antihistamines. Another wise alternative is the liquorice root, since "it increases the amount of naturally generated steroids in your body." It will also help to release the mucus, meaning you can breathe better and cough less, although to validate this, more testing is required.An element that can kill the liver and lungs is found in certain butterbur posts. Butterbur may trigger a reaction if you're allergic to marigolds, ragweed, or daisies.Of diligence, also using licorice. Elevated blood pressure & cardiac problems can be triggered by drinking large quantities. Liqueur additives can bc discouraged for breastfeeding mothers. They can cause preterm labor.

Dietary Changes

Have you ever seen how the nose tends to run when a plate of hot wings is full? That's how salty, hot foods that can help clear nasal passages have an impact.

Add spicy ginger, cayenne pepper, or fenugreek, an herb grown in Asia and Europe, to your meals. It can also help ease your sore nose & un-stuff garlic and onions into your brain, just not as fiery.

4.3Anxiety

As a cure for anxiety, several herbal medications have been tested, but further study is required to explain the dangers and benefits. What we understand & don't know is this:

Kava has proved to be a potential anxiety medication. However, a history of serious liver injury, including with short-term usage, prompted the F.D.A. to provide recommendations on the use of kava-containing dietary supplements. While these initial liver toxicity findings have been questioned, if you are contemplating utilizing items involving kava, take special care and include a doctor in the decision.

A few small research studies show that the passionflower can intensify distress. In several commercial items, passion flowers are mixed with other plants, rendering it difficult to discern the distinctive features of each genus. When consumed as prescribed, passionflower is usually considered healthy, although some reports have shown it can induce drowsiness, dizziness, and confusion.

Individuals that used valerian reported less fear and pressure in several trials. People have reported no advantages in other tests. Valerian is widely thought to be safe at recommended levels, although it is not used for more than a few weeks at a time and, unless approved by the doctor, long-term safety tests are incomplete. It is possible to induce certain unpleasant effects, such as migraine headaches, drowsiness, and dizziness.

Chamomile

Research reveals that chamomile is normally deemed healthy for short-term usage and can be effective in decreasing anxiety symptoms. However, when combined with blood-thinning drugs, chamomile may raise the likelihood of bleeding. The usage of chamomile in certain people that are sensitive to the plant family that includes chamomile, which triggers allergic reactions. Ragweed's, daisies, marigolds, and chrysanthemums are additional representatives of this genus.

Lavender

Many findings indicate that anxiety may be reduced by oral lavender or lavender aromatherapy, however minimal and preliminary study is being done. Oral lavender can induce headaches and constipation. Appetite can also rise, sedative properties of some drugs and vitamins can strengthen, and low blood pressure can be induced.

Balm with Lemon

Preliminary research suggests that some symptoms of fear, such as nervousness & excitability, may be minimized with a lemon balm. Lemon balm is usually well-tolerated for short-term usage and is deemed healthy, but may induce nausea and abdominal pain.

The F.D.A. does not govern herbal products the same way as drugs do. The consistency of such supplements may also be a challenge, considering the improved quality management regulations in effect since 2010. Bear in mind; security doesn't mean usual at all.

Call your doctor first if you are contemplating taking some herbal supplements as an anxiety medication, especially if you are taking other medicines. Severe harmful effects may be induced by the use of certain natural ingredients and some medications.

Any herbal supplements used for anxiety may cause you to feel tired, so they may not be healthy to take while driving or doing risky activities. If you want to pursue herbal supplements, your doctor will advise you to consider the potential dangers and benefits.

If regular tasks are fucked up by fear, speak to the doctor. For symptoms to escalate, more severe cases of depression typically need psychiatric attention or therapeutic intervention (psychotherapy).

4.4 Diarrhea

Diarrhea is triggered more often than not by mild bouts of diet-borne illness or food poisoning. Often, certain infections may be caused by moderate diarrhea.

Using so much food, such as new fruit, consuming foods that you are resistant to or intolerant of, such as milk goods, or developing digestive problems, such as colitis and irritable bowel syndrome, are other sources of diarrhea.

When the large intestine and colon require food waste to travel rapidly, it does not hold moisture and nutrients. The colon will most also draw water from the body and allow it to get rid of extra feces in a rush. Without vital nutrients, all of them will leave them dehydrated.

Astringent herbs:

The intestinal mucous membranes are helped by astringent herbs such as blackberry leaf or raspberry leaf to "dry up" per cup, using one heaping tsp. Drink about half a cup each hour. There is some debate about utilizing these teas while breastfeeding.

Carob powder can be broken down into an industrial replenishing beverage high in fiber (hydrating electrolyte). DO NOT offer a carob to children as told by the doctor to do so.

In the Bilberry extract, the astringent feature is also present (Vaccinium myrtillus). Do not use blackberry if anticoagulants are taken (blood thinners). Theoretically, it is even possible to connect Bilberry to diabetes drugs.

Agrimony is a popular diarrhea treatment. Agrimony may have a blood-thinning effect and can boost the strain in the blood. If you are concerned with these health issues, speak to the doctor before starting agricultural medicine.

Inflammation Reducers:

A fruit-dependent flavonoid, Quercetin, can help reduce inflammation.

Chamomile is commonly taken as a tea (Matricaria recutita). In people that are allergic to ragweed, chamomile can interact with hormone therapies that can cause symptoms.

As a cold-water drink, Althea officinalis (marshmallow root) should be taken. Just digest some root in 1 quart of water pressure overnight. Consume the mix throughout the day. Marshmallow may interact with some drugs, such as lithium, that are administered by mouth. Ulmus fulva or Althaea Officinalis (slippery elm powder) can soothe the intestines (marshmallow root powder). Render a paste with the powder & a lesser volume. Pour in much of the water steadily and then simmer down to one pint. Slippery elm has a well-known reputation for the promotion of rape. It will mess some drugs with it.

Combatants of infection:

Berberine-containing plants can help to treat infectious diarrhea. They include Barberry (Berberis vulgaris), Hydrastis Canadensis (goldenseal), and Berberis aquifolium (Oregon grape). You should NOT take Berberine while you are pregnant or are breastfeeding. Second, consult the doctors if you are taking those prescribed medications.

Representative Bulk-forming:

Psyllium is a soluble fiber that comes from Plantago ovate beans' husks that can help treat diarrhea. It is a bulk-forming agent that serves to stabilize the feces, soaking urine out from the colon. For a high volume of water, take psyllium. Before taking psyllium, people with inflammatory bowel disease should talk to their clinicians.

Be mindful that while doctors with diarrhea can profit from fiber agents such as psyllium, they are most commonly used as a laxative to alleviate constipation. Before using psyllium to treat diarrhea, talk to the doctor.

Homeopathy

Any evidence suggests that diarrhea may be helped by homeopathic care. Children with severe diarrhea who underwent individualized homeopathic medication for five days in one study had substantially less time-consuming diarrhea than children getting a placebo. Homeopaths recognize the constitutional form of an organism in administering a cure, including the physical, behavioral, & intellectual makeup. In deciding on the most fitting solution for a single person, a professional homeopath discusses all of these variables. Any of the most efficient homeopathic procedures include: Arsenicum's Song. For foul-smelling diarrhea and burning pains in the abdomen and around the anus by food poisoning/diarrhea. For individuals who are exhausted and restless & whose symptoms appear to worsen in the cold and strengthen with sunshine, this therapy is more successful. Vomiting can occur as well. In order to avoid diarrhea while traveling, you can also use Arsenicum.

Chamomilla. A glossy greenish stool that smells like rotten eggs. Used for infants, in particular, especially those that are argumentative, irritable, and difficult to console. Chamomile is widely prescribed for colicky or teething infants by clinicians.

Calcarea Carbonica. For teens who dread being isolated or in the dark and who sweat excessively when asleep. The stools may have a rotten odor.

Concerning Mercurius. Used of foul-smelling diarrhea, followed by blood traces, or may provide an incomplete emptying sensation. For people that appear to be slow during bowel motions, undergo drastic changes in body temperature, perspire continuously, and have a thirst for cool drinks, this drug is especially efficient.

Podophyllum. Gushing, explosive, painless diarrhea, which gets worse after consuming or eating. Sometimes, exhaustion accompanies bowel movements. In the lower extremities, the person for whom this drug is appropriate can suffer painful cramps. For diarrhea suffered by teething, clinicians can use podophyllum in infants.

Sulfur. For weepy, irritable teenagers. With the odor of rotten eggs, they can get diarrhea and a red ring around the anus.

Veratrum's song. Exhaustion, sore stomach, cough, chills, diarrhea that is profuse and watery, abdominal cramps.

The diarrhea is exacerbated by fruit, and the patient craves good liquids.

Acupuncture

While several reports have reported progress in the treatment of childhood diarrhea in the journals of Traditional Chinese Medicine, acupuncturists in the United States do not treat this disorder commonly in infants. Acupuncture can, therefore, be discovered after traditional treatment has collapsed. In this situation, acupuncturists look at the consistency of nutrition as well as the "energetic" qualities of food that may hinder digestion.

When managing diarrhea in adults, acupuncture is often combined with traditional medicine.

Centered on an individualized analysis of qi excesses and defects found in several meridians, Acupuncturists treat diarrhea patients. In the case of diarrhea, Qi dysfunction of the meridian of the spleen is generally found. As a consequence, therapies for acupuncture also depend on reinforcing this meridian. Acupuncturists also make use of moxibustion.

4.5Asthma

Natural Treatment Treatments Cure Asthma

You already realize that pharmaceutical medications are the greatest medication expense linked to asthma, whether you have asthma or concern about someone who does. Asthma treatment in the United States costs $6 billion a year, according to the A.L.A. (American Lung Association).

Keeping track with multiple inhalers and drugs may also be a pain, in addition to the cost of asthma medicines. You may be worried about finding an herbal remedy or holistic treatment for your asthma whether you are searching for safe sources of asthma care or looking for ways to strengthen your asthma symptom management.

A variety of individuals with asthma are pursuing alternative therapy in order to enhance their asthma symptom regulation.

Most individuals use alternative therapies, especially for allergic diseases.

For about 40 % of people with the condition of allergy are currently looking for a natural cure. "In accordance with conventional (treatment), often persons utilize it."

However, what does the study reveal regarding herbal treatments, and why do individuals owe them a shot? "Some of these have demonstrated advantages in animals as being anti-inflammatory," but in human trials, sadly, they have not really been proven to be successful.

While steam baths (warm) have also been used to aid relieve asthma-related nasal inflammation and airway pressure, it is pointed out that there has never been proof that steam therapies may ease asthma symptoms. It is important to remember that this is not a treatment for asthma. And still, just because the study has not identified a definitive advantage doesn't mean that many individuals won't benefit from steam baths.

'Steam baths' can ease any of the effects as they provide the airways with moisture. Nevertheless, they warn that steam may be dangerously hot, "However, they caution that steam may be dangerously hot,"

Steam baths can help to compensate for some symptoms, especially stuffiness of the nasal, but baths of steam are not "a replacement for medications of asthma."

Herbs & other asthma alternative treatment options

A variety of herbs have been reported as natural asthma remedies, but it is recommended that when taking these asthma medications, individuals should be vigilant. These alternate therapeutic approaches and the related risks and incentives include:

Garlic.

Thanks to its anti-inflammatory effects, garlic is used as a natural medication to treat many illnesses, especially heart disease. Since asthma disease is inflammatory, it might seem sensible that garlic might also be helpful in relieving the symptoms of asthma. However, it is reported that no laboratory studies have been undertaken exploring the impact of garlic on the symptoms of asthma. Hence, its function remains unclear in the management of asthma. However, the usage of garlic as an additional option for asthma is also being checked.

Ginger

It is also known to ease inflammation, and a new report has found that oral ginger extracts are associated with improving the symptoms of asthma. However, the research did not indicate that ginger application contributed to any real change in lung function. It is therefore advised that this research be used as an alternative therapy for asthma to draw certain assumptions regarding the application of ginger. Further experiments are also being carried out in order to assess more closely whether or not ginger can regulate the effects of asthma more effectively.

Echinacea & the Licorice Root.

One research investigating the usage of a variety of various herbs to combat asthma showed that not only was Echinacea, an herb frequently used to treat infections of upper respiratory, unsuccessful, but it was also correlated with a variety of side effects. The complications involved with the usage of Echinacea are worsening asthma, skin rashes & potential liver damage when combined with other drugs. Likewise, it has been found that licorice leaves, which have antioxidant and anti-inflammatory properties and are often used by people with asthma to soothe their lungs, are inadequate as a potential cure for asthma and are also correlated with adverse results such as high blood pressure. No clinical tests have proven that both Echinacea and licorice root are an effective treatment for asthma and there have been several findings that in some people, Echinacea may worsen symptoms of asthma.

Turmeric.

Turmeric has been the focus of a variety of experiments, and some anti-allergy properties have been identified. It is assumed that turmeric, which may induce inflammation, has an effect on histamines. However, before Turmeric can be identified as a safe and efficient natural treatment for asthma, more research must be performed.

Honey.

Honey, used to help soothe an irritated throat & calm a cough, is an ingredient of many cold and cough remedies. There is no evidence to support its use as an alternative therapy for asthma symptoms, although many people with asthma may try to blend honey with a hot drink for relaxation.

Omega-3s

Omega-3 fatty acids are also used as a natural therapy to effectively avoid and cure cardiovascular disease. Although some literature shows that omega-3s may also help minimize inflammation of the airway and improve lung capacity, there is still a great deal that is not understood regarding their role in the treatment of asthma.

4.6Bites and Stings

With all its majesty, summer is here, and for plenty of us, it means more time spent outdoors. Like every gardener or outdoor enthusiast acknowledges, once you have an unexpected encounter with insect bites or stings, it is usually only a matter of time. The outcome may differ from mild pain to disease or even death. Mosquitos, mosquitoes, black flies, fleas, bees, horse flies, chiggers, and deer flies are the most popular biting or stinging species.

A safer alternative to insecticides, which can include substances such as DEET & permethrin and may cause harmful consequences for many, can be natural remedies.

An ounce of security is worth a pound of medication, "An ounce of protection is worth a pound of treatment," For their insect-repellent qualities, some essential oils (plants) are beneficial. Pennyroyal, citronella, cedarwood, cinnamon leaf oil, eucalyptus, & catnip oil are a few of the more popular. In order to create a bug spray, these can be applied to water. Notice that pregnant mothers should stop utilizing Pennyroyal. Alternatively, there are available widely distributed citronella candles.

When you try your utmost to hold pests at bay, but always end up with a burn or scrape, relaxing pain and curing the face are the primary objectives. In this case, the following herbs can be useful.

Mentha piperita (Peppermint)

Through cooling the peppermint oil and crushed leaves, it will soothe itchy or sore bites.

Plantago Major (Plantain)

For mosquito bites, fresh plantain leaves could be used. New plantain leaves may be combined with bentonite clay & water in order to produce a paste to make a poultice. A leaf can, instead, be chewed and put right over the bite.

Calendula officinalis (calendula)

Calendula oil and fresh leaves can soothe bruised, itchy skin and will guarantee quick healing of bites and stings. With calendula, beeswax, & antiseptic essential oils, such as rosemary, tea tree, and lavender, a simple salve can be grown.

Symphytum officinale (Comfrey)

For different skin disorders, including rashes, scrapes, and bruises, Comfrey enriched oil or fresh leaf juice may be used topically. It can relieve itching and discomfort linked to bites and stings.

Hamamelissa (Witch Hazel)

Witch hazel distillate is commonly available in supermarkets, and for mild skin irritations, it is an over-the-counter relief. Integrate three components of baking soda into 1.5 components of witch hazel to make an itch-soothing potion.These drugs are produced from plants & ingredients that are easily found. A few (or all) on hand are wise, particularly in the summer months, when bites, stings, bruises, and scrapes eventually happen.

4.7Bronchitis, Cold Chest, and Pneumonia

Hot Treatments for Normal Bronchitis, Pneumonia, and Chest The plurality of individuals gets a common cough. However, it ends in a respiratory condition known as bronchitis, and this simple cough is followed by serious symptoms such as breathlessness & phlegm. A cough or fever also weakens the immune system, and people are therefore at increased risk of contracting bronchitis. Persistent bronchitis may contribute to asthma & chronic obstructive pulmonary disease (C.O.P.D.), and if not managed, it may be life-threatening. Much like any other condition, bronchitis may also be divided into severe or recurrent. Inflamed or enlarged bronchial tubes that hold oxygen between the lungs, mouth, and nose. For anyone diagnosed with bronchitis, it is rather difficult to inhale air into the lungs. A frequent source of bronchitis is inhaling toxic gases and air containing pollen. For certain individuals suffering with bronchitis, inhaling contaminated air may be worse. In reality, smoking is believed to be the primary cause of bronchitis and smokers are at a greater risk of contracting this disease. This is because cigarettes release different chemicals and the lining of the bronchial tube or surface is disturbed as individuals inhale these chemicals. For this reason, they get recurrent bronchitis. Smoking induces cells to grow more mucus than usual, allowing the bronchial tubes to become inflamed. This mucus has the potential to coat the whole bronchial lining as well, contributing to the accumulation of bronchitis-causing contagious bacteria. This worsens the condition of the person suffering from bronchitis. Signs of bronchitis include phlegm or dry cough, fever, shortness of breath, and fatigue sometimes.Home remediation to relieve bronchitis-induced inflammation

1. Saunth (dry ginger), Pipli (long pepper), & Kali Mirch (black pepper)

In the event of swelling bronchial passages, Saunth has anti-inflammatory properties that offer relief. In helping to get rid of nasal inflammation, Kali Mirch is truly successful. Long pepper, or pipli, is well recognized for its anti-inflammatory effects. Ayurveda specialist B N Sinha recommends that all three components be combined with honey in powdered form and that the mixture be eaten for immediate results three times a day.

2. Juice of Giloy

Giloy (Tinospora Cordifolia) is an herb which was used and changed in the medicine of Indian for decades, derived from Ayurveda. On the lining of the neck, Giloy has a supportive cushion and hence allows the inflamed bronchial lining to offer relief. For relaxation, consume the juice once in the morning and once in the evening.

3. The Water that is Warm

Increase the absorption of water and limit yourself to consuming just hot water. It will help to decrease lung swelling and soothe the track. Sometimes, physicians prescribe improved water consumption following a bacterial cough and a cold.

4. Soup of Tomato

Apart from becoming a winter reliever, tomato soup is extremely high in vitamin C, which tends to prevent prolonged mucus production in the midst of bronchitis. Only consume tomato soup twice a day, at the very least. Put some freshly ground pepper on top to make tomato soup, so it becomes a sumptuous meal that is safe, wholesome, and extremely good for you.

5. Trikatu and the Garlic Powder

It is recommended to mix and dry four parts of garlic powder and one part of trikatu, plus a small amount of honey, twice a day. Although garlic in any kitchen is a popular ingredient, it was highly prized in ancient times for its numerous health-beneficial properties that are still followed today in many cultures.

6. Broth of ginger

Ginger, especially in Ayurveda healing, has numerous advantages. Ginger has characteristics that are very good in cough therapy. If it is not ginger soup, you may drink ginger tea, which is just as effective. The ginger powder is obtained from the ginger root, which is ground. It is a thin off-white substance with a potent fragrance and a pungent flavor, or more brownish.

7. Massaging of Mustard Oil

Mustard oil is reddish-brown/amber and comes from mustard seeds (black, white, and brown). It has been widely used since ancient times in eastern and northern India and comes with a bevy of beneficial effects. A soft mustard oil massage helps bring relief from a sore chest. The inflammation in the lungs is relieved by massaging with mustard oil. People suffering from bronchitis are recommended, apart from these quick and easy to reach home remedies, to avoid curd & other cold items that can aggravate the disease. Keep warm as humans, especially during the winter months, are more vulnerable to cold and cough spells. When one is prone to coughing and cold allergies, smoke must be stopped.

4.8Sunburns and Burns

Sunburns arise periodically, sometimes among the most vigilant of wearers of sunscreen. Luckily, there are a host of common ways to treat a burn at home by utilizing products that you might already have on your bathroom shelf or in your refrigerator.

1. Aloe Vera

Aloe Vera gel can do more than offer soothing skin relief, probably one of the most common sunburn treatment techniques. The gel also has anti-inflammatory properties that can help sunburned skin relax. This summer, hold the bottle of aloe vera in the travel bag or, even cooler, just use the plant gel and apply it when appropriate.

2. Hyaluronic acid

"It is suggested that you apply a facial cream packed with hyaluronic acid "to help the skin heal faster." Hyaluronic acid can moisturize & plump solar-parched skin without creating more discomfort as a hydrating agent created naturally by the body.

3. White Vinegar

Doctors are recommending the addition of white vinegar to the infected regions for burning discomfort and annoyance. "It may help alleviate discomfort and irritation and function as an antiseptic since white vinegar is made of acetic acid,"

4. Baking Soda

The normal pH degree of your skin is another key factor to be taken into consideration when managing sunburn at home. It is recommended to create a cold compress composed of baking soda & water to help stabilize the pH of burnt skin and apply it for fifteen minutes to sunburned skin.

5. Leaf Tea Around

Compared to baking soda compresses, since they produce polyphenols that are anti-inflammatory, it is better to give green tea compresses a try. Just steep green tea leaves & a clean soaked rag soak the steep tea. Enable the compress to cool for 15 minutes in the refrigerator until the compress is added to the sunburned face.

6. Greece's yogurt

Greek yogurt has anti-inflammatory properties attributable to lactic acid which can be used to soothe and moisturize sunburned skin. "Greek yogurt is strained more often than traditional yogurt [and] is, therefore, thicker & has a greater concentration of probiotics," "Current findings have shown that topical probiotic treatment improves the irritation and redness of the skin." Pure, organic Greek yogurt can be applied to the body and face as a mask and rinsed after fifteen minutes with Greek yogurt to soothe the sunburn.

4.9Fever

This natural treatments would help you to stay calm and comfortable if you are coping with a low temperature.

If your forehead feels feverish, you should search for acetaminophen (Tylenol) or ibuprofen (Advil) to decrease the temperature.

But don't be scared to let it run its course whether the fever is 101 °F (38.3 ° C) or below. However, if you're uncomfortable and want to take steps, consider some home cure remedies that will help tame the flames.

How to calm the fever

Soak yourself in a lukewarm bath. If you have a headache, this temperature will sound good enough and the bath can help lower the body temperature. Through falling into icy temperatures, you don't want to immediately put down a fever; the treatment sends blood racing to tissues (internal), which is how the body protects itself against ice. Instead of cooling down, the interior actually warms up.

A sponge bath is probable. Sponging high-heat areas with cold water such as the armpits & groin will help decrease the temperature as water evaporation begins.

Place cool & damp washcloths on the forehead & back of the neck while you're not cleaning.

Drink a little tea

Brew the yarrow tea in a cup. This herb expands the lungs and causes the process of sweating that brings a fever to an end. Steep a tablespoon of the herb for 10 minutes in a cup of freshly distilled water. Just let cool it. Before you begin sweating, drink one or two cups.

Another vine, the elderflower, is also enhanced by sweat. And it appears to be helpful for some flu-related complications and colds, such as mucus overproduction. Mix up 2 tsp. Create the elderflower tea from the herb in a cup of boiling water and let it steep for 15 mins. Strain the elderflower down with it. Drink until the fever lasts, three times a day. Elderberries are also rich in antioxidant-creating immunity.

Drink a cup of hot tea with ginger, which often triggers transpiration. To create the tea, brew a half-tsp of minced ginger root in a cup of just-boiled water. Uh, strain. Drink afterward.

Willow bark can help ease a headache and is a good Aspirin alternative. Consume it in a powdered form, as a tincture, or even as a tea.

Get it spicy

Sprinkle cayenne pepper on the diet while you have a fever. Capsaicin, the alarmingly hot compound that's used in hot peppers, is one of the key ingredients. Cayenne helps you sweat and promotes fast blood flow as well.

Get your socks wet

Try a wet sock cure for fever, a common household medication. Warm your foot in a warm bath first. So, wash a pair of thin socks of cotton in cold water, rinse them, and put them on before you head to bed. Place the socks pair over the ones that are wet (dry wool). By carrying blood to the foot, this procedure tends to reduce a fever, which greatly improves blood circulation.

A mustard foot bath is another route for the foot to collect blood. Add 2 tsp of mustard powder to four cups of hot water in a tub large enough for one's feet, and soak.

Keep calm about it

For curing a fever, an old folk cure is to wash a towel in cool water and cover yourself in it. Today, physicians warn you not to lower your body temperature too soon, so if you are pursuing this method, choose water that is mildly damp, not cold. Cover the saturated sheet with a wide blanket or beach towel and lay down for about fifteen minutes. When the damp sheet continues to get wet, unwrap yourself.

Drink beverages

When one has a fever, it is easy to become dehydrated. Drink 8 to 12 glasses of water a day, or enough to render your pee pale. Having a sporting drink like Gatorade may also be helpful. It restores not only fluids that have been lost to dehydration, but also minerals that have been lost.

Orange juice and other vitamin C-rich fruit juices are healthier options since vitamin C allows the immune system to avoid infection.

Cool grapes give a soothing incentive and hydration.

4.10Dyspepsia, Indigestion

Indigested causes

Indigestion is also caused by overeating, chewing too hard, or drinking too much greasy or hot food. Indigestion can also be caused by these psychological conditions, including depression or anxiety.

In individuals with the following disorders, indigestion can be more frequent:

- Ulcers peptics
- Pancreatitis.
- G.R.E.D.
- Disease in the breast
- Anomaly in the bile ducts or pancreas
- Gallstones
- Gastritis.

For Natural Treatments

While there is little literature on natural indigestion cures, peppermint tea or consuming ginger can be prescribed by alternative medicine practitioners to ease the digestive tract after a meal.

Studies indicate that certain other herbal therapies can provide indigestion relief as well:

Extract of the Leaf for Artichoke

Artichoke is rich in antioxidants & antimicrobial properties and is popular in Mediterranean countries. It has been used to prevent liver injury, decrease cholesterol levels and manage dyspepsia.

A 2015 study tracked men and women aged 17 to 80 years who suffered from stomach discomfort or vomiting in the case of nausea or bloating over a span of three months. Since drinking a supplementary blend of artichoke leaf extract and ginger for around two weeks, only the group who consumed the blend felt a reduction in symptoms. Researchers noticed at four weeks that in more than 60 percent of cases, the medication minimized indigestion. They theorized that the antispasmodic effects of artichoke leaf extract and its capacity to facilitate bile acid secretion also assist gastrointestinal transit, helping to relieve bloating and fullness.

Peppermint and Caraway Oil

Research has shown that products made up of a combination of enteric-coated peppermint oil and caraway oil can help ease indigestion symptoms. It is believed that the muscles of the stomach will relax this formula and let food flow quicker through the stomach.

Indications

Although the hallmark of indigestion is stomach discomfort during a meal, other signs may include:

- Nausea
- Epigastric burning or pain, moderate to intolerable (located between the bones of the chest (lower end & navel)
- Belching
- Bloating

Since indigestion in some cases may suggest a more serious infection, it is necessary to seek medical treatment if you have symptoms such as:

- Desperately swallowing
- Regularly vomiting
- Decrease of weight or lack of appetite
- Bloody or black stool
- Sweating indigestion, shortness of breath, or pain that radiates to the throat, mouth, or arm
- Heartburn new or irritated

Remedies Using Herbs

It is too early to prescribe some natural medicines as a remedy for indigestion, owing to inadequate studies. It is, therefore, necessary to remember that a condition's self-management and the dismissal or discontinuation of routine care may have vital implications. Be sure to contact the doctor first if you are considering the use of herbal medication in indigestion care.

It can help to decrease the risk of indigestion by actually slowing down while you eat. These preventive methods involve minimizing the consumption of caffeine and carbonated beverages, utilizing calming approaches such as deep relaxation & meditation, instead of two to three bigger meals, and preparing fewer, more frequent meals.

Normal indigestion remedies involve antacids or drugs that suppress acid output or allow the stomach to move food into the small intestine more effectively.

Conclusion

Native Americans have played a vital role in making us realize that how important herbalism. The medicinal & herbal wisdom of the Native Americans has been overlooked by history for so long. This book aims to introduce their medicinal experience and deep knowledge of natural supplements back to life.

With this book on the shelves, you have at your hands a proud tradition of herbal craftsmanship & herbal culture. You have covered all the little details about how to grow the herbs in your backyard. Moreover, the use of the most important herbs, natural remedies, and supplements of the herbs in the local market is also part of the book

Carry it along in the walks of nature: this book will lead you through the method of identification, wildcrafting, & even transplanting herbs that are commonly found, yet woefully disregarded, in your own yard.

In your path to becoming a conscientious, compassionate, and qualified herbalist, this handy encyclopedia will lead you from the ground to the table. Enjoy reading this book and learn as much as you can about this beautiful gift of nature known as herbs or plants.

NATIVE AMERICAN HERBAL DISPENSATORY

The Ultimate Herbal Dispensatory to Discover the Secrets and Forgotten Practices of Native American Herbal Medicine

Introduction

For decades, Native American herbal medicines have been used to treat chronic diseases and cure diverse health problems. Native Americans depended on the many plants that flourished near their homes, as they have no access to physicians or hospitals. Most of this knowledge has been forgotten; there are, however, some that continue to record the remaining recipes. Native American herbal medicines are still being used to treat numerous illnesses today. However, before trying any herbal cure, you need to study the particular remedy and speak to your health care provider. Native Americans were as vulnerable as anybody else to respiratory problems. Teas derived from natural ingredients or blends of these ingredients were used to treat allergies, coughs and colds. To loosen and remove phlegm, they treated asthma with skunk cabbage. For bronchitis, pneumonia, and other respiratory ailments, the pleurisy root was used. It is also an exceptional cure for these diseases. Wormwood has also been prescribed for multiple bronchitis conditions. For the discomfort of colds and flu, Sage was used. The tribes used the boneset to cure coughs and colds. To treat the cold, a similar aspen tea was prepared from the Aspen tree's inner bark.

For the same reason, Wild Cherry tea, produced from the bark of the Wild Cherry Tree, was also made into tea. Likewise, as a cough syrup, sarsaparilla was mixed with the sweet flag. Rabbit tobacco and Bloodroot were similarly used to relieve different effects of cold, cough and flu. To get relief from back pain, they used arnica as a rub or a poultice. Also, horsemint tea was drunk to deal with back pains. Under the harsh conditions under which many tribes existed, diarrhea may easily cause dehydration. When stomach problems arose, these Native American herbal medicines were used. Unless otherwise noted, these treatments were used in tea form.

Diarrhea

- Black cherry root
- Dogwood bark tea is used as enemas.
- Black Raspberry root
- Black cherry fruit was fermented naturally for up to a year. Finally, the juice was used to cure dysentery.

Other Digestive Disorders

- Dandelion roots were used to treat urinary tract problems and heartburn.

- Yellow Root was used as a cure for stomach related issues.
- Sage was used to treat stomach problems.
- Juniper was used to cure urinary tract infections.
- Juniper was also used to treat diarrhea.
- Elder was used as a laxative.

To get relief from menstrual cramps, provide ease in childbirth, remedy hormonal imbalances, and fix libido disorders, Wild Yam root was used very effectively. They used sage in a particular manner to manage irregular menstruation, childbirth-related complications and bleeding.

Passion Flower was used for:

- Tension
- Insomnia
- Earache

They used willow to treat:

- Pain
- Fever

- Headache

Purple Coneflower was used to cure:

- Snakebite
- Insect bites
- Toothaches

They used Black Cohosh to manage and treat the following issues:

- Female hormones
- Tinnitus
- Sciatica
- Arthritis
- Cough
- Headaches

Skullcap was used to treat:

- Restless leg
- Nervous tension
- Insomnia

The herbal medicines that the Native Americans used to cure many diseases are still being grown, gathered and produced by many Native Americans. Many of the popular natural medicines you find are before Native American treatments in your local health food store. Many of those herbs used by the Native Americans were given for their diseases to early settlers. For centuries, these herbs have been used, and many were in traditional medicinal usage before the advent of mainstream medicines. Any of the choices for capsules and tinctures we have were not available to Native Americans. It's more than probable that much of their herbal medicines were made into teas. Modern types of these herbs have the same function and work as tea in many cases. This book contains several remedies and preparation techniques to help you naturally treat different sicknesses.

Native American Medicine

Through a powerful oral tradition, Native Americans' generations have obtained medical information over the past 40,000 years. The interconnection between humanity, ecology, and the spiritual realm is emphasized by indigenous medical philosophy. A person of medicine studies the relationships of the patient with other individuals, the individual's physical well-being, and establishes a holistic approach for healing. A combination of therapies and experiences are used to treat and cure the patient. These may include herbs, ceremony, music, prayer and sweating.

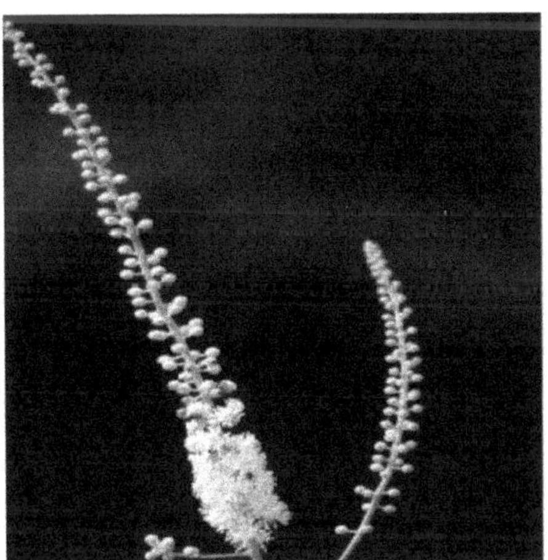

To cure cardiovascular disorders and many other cancers and diseases, black cohosh, a traditional medicinal herb, was used. The effectiveness of Native American medical therapies is now accepted by western medicine. Traditional and new medicines are not inherently mutually exclusive. Thus they can be used in concert with each other. Any of the plants used by Native American physicians can now be found in commercial stores around the country. They include black cohosh that is used to treat cardiovascular issues. Similarly, Echinacea is used to cure infections.

Native American Medicine History

Native American medicine relates to over 500 nations' combined clinical practices. Native medicine is almost forty thousand years old. The particular activities differed between tribes, but everything is based on the universal idea that man is an integral part of nature and that a matter of balance is health. When interrelationships are valued, nurtured and sustained in harmony, the natural world then moves as a consequence. The natural world cannot be seen by the mind and does not engage in science directly and intuitively. Much like a human being's inner life cannot be determined, nature has persuasive forces that need to be incorporated for balance. Just now has reporting started and has been limited to findings, so it is incomplete. Native medicine values all life and is not just a body of science or methodology that is scholarly.

For fear of exploitation, Native American elders typically do not disclose their knowledge.

The balance between the inner life and open actions is tackled in Native American medicine. They all take into account the body, mind, soul, thoughts, social circle and lifestyle. The choice and desires of a patient are often respected to establish harmony. Bodywork, naturopathy, bone setting, midwifery, hydrotherapy, botanical, and nutritional medicine can be included in every Native American healer's strategy. Often used are ceremonial and ritual medicines. Many of this has been forgotten as only by living practitioners has this undocumented living practice survived. More Native Americans have been involved in protecting their culture, and Native American medicine today is as fluid as ever with this effort.

1.1 The Treatment approach

Native American medicine is a complete framework that balances every sphere of one's life, including lifestyle and social interactions with one inner world. Native medicine assumes that in the divine realm, the roots of every imbalance lie. In the course of every recovery procedure, spiritual approaches are vital. Including fees and rates, clinical approaches are often clearly and uniquely tailored for the patient. They require, as part of the healing method, the process of fee negotiation. The Healing Elder seems to have the most healing strength, and the elder practitioner loses his prestige as a powerful healer when treatment fails. The person in need of healing makes a proposition to the doctor of medicine and waits to see if it is approved. Face-to-face, they rarely negotiate. The customer leaves the bid outside the healer's door, and if it remains there till the morning, it means that it has not been approved, and one can go somewhere. Once they understand, therapy will, for example, start with a behavioral prescription, a pledge, a selfless act, genuine repentance, or scaling a holy mountain. Techniques include self-inquiry and discovery to ascertain whether there is a need for a dietary improvement, prayer, herbs, massage, a sweat lodge ritual or a vision quest.

1.2 Theories

The main objective is to alter the patient's comprehension of the world through a healthier self-concept, increased acceptance of others and behavior adjustments. The healer's goal is not only to treat sickness but to change the patient's overall approach towards life and the world around him. Native American medicine combines science as well as spirit with the onset of new technology. They mostly use herbal interventions and pharmaceuticals. We can explain this by narrating a Native American story on the use of herbal medicine. Barb, a wife, mother and lawyer, is still fighting breast cancer. She did what she could normally do, and the cancer continued to spread despite all her efforts. She met with an Indian elder named Big Nose in a sweat lodge. He wanted to understand what she was doing or what hadn't changed in her life. Deep inside, as a mother-wife and lawyer, she thought she was a loser, and now she's healing herself. It was the pessimistic self-talk that needed to end, Big Nose told her. Barb decided to let go of her arrogant thought that she would be cured and started to enjoy the moment with her family due to this relationship. There is another story that talks of a woman who had had extreme arthritis. She was desperately looking for the right healer. To facilitate recovery, medicine men go further and beyond the current problem and understand radical improvement is often required. The shifts are primary, and herbs are secondary, along with massage and prayer. Right relationships, the correction of relationships with oneself, families, members of the society and the spiritual environment are all effects of disruption of relationships and disease development.

Training

Native American healers, through apprenticeships, educate their students. For preparation, several weeks of testing the purpose and dedication of a student are vital. An apprentice gains patience and respect and acquires knowledge. Native medicine is still an oral tradition. It cannot be taught in an academic setting. Students may learn the skills required only by experience, and only when the patient is ready does the older instructor encourage them to begin a medical practice.

The Main Role of Ceremonies

A crucial aspect of traditional aboriginal healing is the ritual. Due to the close relationship between physical & spiritual well-being, body and soul should heal together. Popular healing rituals encourage well-being by representing ancestral concepts of the world, creator, and spirit. Prayer, drumming, chants, poems, legends & the use of several religious artifacts may be part of them. Wherever an ill person requires healing, healers can perform ceremonies, but the ceremonies are sometimes performed in sacred places. The special buildings are also mentioned as the Medicine Lodges for healing. Traditional healing rituals are considered holy wherever they take place & are only performed by the native healers & local spiritual facilitators. The Non-Natives can take part only by invitation. Native powwows, on the other hand, have grown today into most social and cultural activities that include indigenous music, singing, drumming, regalia, and food. Most powwows welcome all persons.

The Medicine Wheel and the Four Directions

Medicine Wheel, also referred to as the Holy Hoop, has been used for health and healing by thousands of diverse Native American tribes. Also, Father Heaven, Spirit Tree, and Mother Earth represent the Four Paths, symbolizing the dimensions of well-being and life cycles. There are several different shapes that Medicine Wheel could take. It could be artwork, or a real structure on the ground, such as an artifact or painting. Over the past few decades, hundreds of thousands, even, of the medicine wheels that have been constructed on tribal lands in North America. Movement is circular in Medicine Wheel & in the Native American formalities, & typically in the direction of the clock, or the direction is sun-wise. It tends to sync with nature's powers, like gravity & sun's rising & setting.

1.3 Meanings of the Four Directions

Medicine Wheel is viewed differently by various tribes. Usually, each of the Four Directions (West, East, North and South) is represented by a distinctive hue, such as red, black, yellow, & white, representing human races for some. The Directions may also indicate:

- **Stages of life:** the birth, youth, adulthood (or elder) and death

- **Element of the nature:** sun (or fire), water, earth and air
- **Animals:** Bear, Eagle, Buffalo, Wolf, & many more
- **Seasons of the year:** spring, summer, winter, fall
- **Aspects of life:** spiritual, emotional, intellectual, physical
- **Ceremonial plants:** sweet grass, tobacco,cedar, sage

1.4 Healing Plants

For a broad range of medical uses, Alaska Native, Native American & healers of Native Hawaiian all have a long tradition of using the native or indigenous plants. Medicinal plants are as varied as tribes that use them and their uses. Beyond their medical effects, before Western settlement, native plants were the staple of aboriginal people's diet. Today, the indigenous plant is central to current generations' attempts to enhance nutritional wellbeing. "Waianae Diet" & "Pre-Captain Diet Cook" are trying to decrease fat, empty calories, & additives. At the same time they are trying to facilitate a healthier and diet that is balanced by restoring indigenous foods' role.

1.5 Intersections of Traditional and Western Healing

Today, the issue of either depending on conventional native healing practices or pursuing Western medical care is frequently confronted by Native Americans of both groups. The two cultures existed in tandem relatively until recently, with really no intersections between them. However, now, the continuum of health services can be accessed by Native Americans. Within tribal communities, most traditional healers are still practicing independently. To organize treatment for Native American patients, other healers can collaborate with Western-trained foremost care physicians. Some healthcare facilities, often at the same location, provide both conventional and Western medicine. In certain areas, rather than by tribal health centers or hospitals, patients of Native Americans receive conventional healing from inside the local tribal population. In the Upper Plains Tribes of Lakota and Dakota, & Mandan, Hidatsa, & Arikara, (MHA), tribal member arranges for the services by directly calling nearby healers. Many Western-trained doctors often recommend patients to conventional healers and may sometimes assist a specific patient in coordinating traditional and Western medicine.

Mint and Sage Herbal Remedies

The Mint family's plants resemble with feathers of the birds. Moreover, by observing and comparing them, you can discover that they share the following characteristics:

- Four-Sided Square Stems
- Extremely aromatic (Majority of the mint family plants have a strong aroma)
- Tiny flowers have five united petals (three down, two-up). Together they make upper & lower "lips" which form tubule which is just right for the hummingbirds & butterflies
- Flowers are usually arranged in clusters at leaves' base or end of the spikes
- Nearly 1/2 of the common kitchen's spices are from the mint family

2.1 Mint Family Herbal Medicine

The aromatic essence of the family plants of mint comes from their elevated levels of volatile oils, which also explains for rich flavors & many of the medicinal properties valued in cooking. Although plants of mint family's medicinal actions make a reasonably long list and all of them fall into the categories of four:

- Nervine for complaints affecting the nervous system (depression, anxiety, headaches, dementia, insomnia)

- Digestive for concerns about the digestive system: (gas, indigestion, cramps, colic, nausea)

- Antimicrobials for the infections: (viral, fungal, bacterial)

- Clearing for concerns about the respiratory system (infection, asthma, congestion)

The plants comprise volatile oils, including, but not limited to, thymol, menthol, citronellal, camphor, limonene, carvacrol, & linalool. Aside from antimicrobial behavior, the main action of the volatile oils in our internal organs is to reduce stress and spasm. Our good smell sense is closely associated with the brain's limbic system, regulating feeling and memory. Nerve finishing is activated to transmit signals to the limbic system & to systems that control discomfort in the internal organs when we catch the fragrance of an aromatic plant; as volatile oils reach our blood, muscles that are smooth in airways & circulatory tissues inside the intestines are relaxed, relieving strain & restoring balance. As for nervine effects, feelings of "existing in flow" or sense of equilibrium is mirrored in our mental condition by the relaxed state generated in our internal organs. It is most probable because fresh smells mean a changing atmosphere and behave as a wake-up request, helping us shift from a tense environment to a calmer state. Briefly, the volatile oil is excellent for destroying microorganisms, from microbes and fungi to viruses, concerning the antimicrobial activity of mint family plants. During periods of illness and disease, aromatics were utilized as the strewing herbs inside homes in Middle Ages to fight 'evil,' also known as microorganisms. And as a sinus infection cure, what else could have been more divine than the mint family aromatherapy? The aromatic activity of the plants of the mint family relaxes tissue of the respiratory system & clears the airways, causing congestion to pass out and breathing to flow easily, whether it is a cup of peppermint tea for the nasal congestions, facial steam of thyme for soothing cough, or the hyssop syrup for moving lung congestion.

2.2 The Mint Family Herbal Remedies

Lemon glycerite balm, a bowl of the tabbouleh with the spearmints for lunch, a whiff of lavender essential oil during rush hour traffic, a cup of cool peppermint tea as a midday-afternoon pick-up, calming cup of the catnip tea soon after a meal, or a revitalizing foot soak of lavender essential oil during rush hour traffic, are so many simple ways to incorporate the uplifting, soothing, and tasty essence of mint into your day. Given below are a few quick remedies.

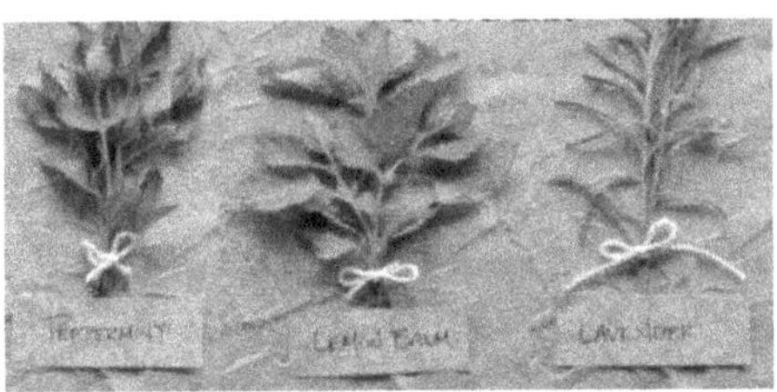

2.3 Peppermint Sun Tea

It is an amazing and excellent recipe for a hot summer day. We have listed below the ingredients that you would require for preparing this Native American herbal recipe:

- Half cup or one cup dried or fresh peppermint leaves.
- Half gallon of tap water.

Given below are the detailed instructions for preparing this Native American herbal recipe. You need to follow these instructions in the given order.

- Put peppermint & water in half a gallon of a glass jar.
- Put in a sunny area for two to eight hours.

- Move to the fridge and let it cool. Enjoy it as a cold drink.

2.4 Tummy Tea

We have listed below the ingredients that you would require for preparing this Native American herbal recipe:

- D Dried chamomile flowers
- catnip leaf, Dried
- lemon balms leaf Dried

Given below are the detailed instructions for preparing this Native American herbal recipe. You need to follow these instructions in the given order.

- Combine equal parts of lemon balm, chamomile and catnip thoroughly in a jar. Then cap & label.
- Then To brew tea, put one tablespoon of the tea blend into eight ounces of water boiled. Then allow it to steep for three to four minutes.
- You can add sweeteners as per your taste, or you may not. Finally enjoy.
- Keep in mind one thing that chamomile will get bitter if it is steeped for a long time.

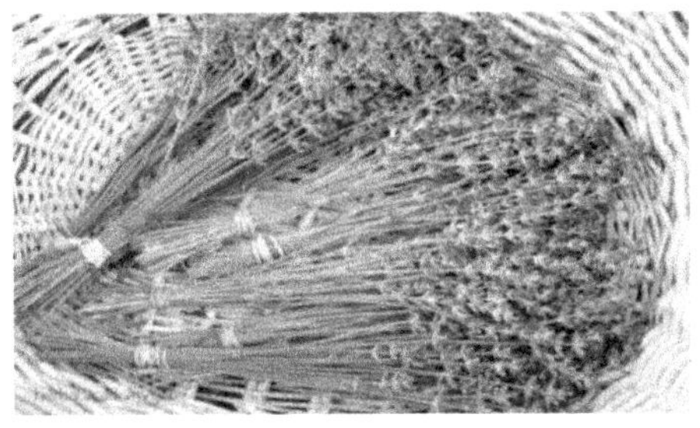

2.5 Lavender Honey

We have listed below the ingredients that you would require for preparing this Native American herbal recipe:

- Fresh or Dried buds of lavender flower
- Local honey, raw

Given below are the detailed instructions for preparing this Native American herbal recipe. You need to follow these instructions in the given order.

- Fill the jar(either half or quarter) with the flower buds. Next, fill it with honey.
- The air bubbles should be removed by poking with a knife or chopstick. Then mix well.
- Allow the mixture to infuse for a week or month, depends on the preferred strength. You need to taste it occasionally till it's suited perfectly to taste buds.

2.6 Sage and Honey Cough Syrup

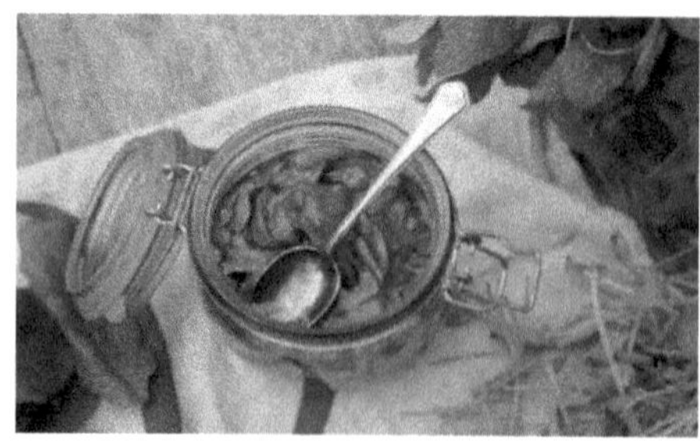

The majority of the people do not like to take medicine. Much of the medicine that we need is given by nature. Now we're going to teach you how to make a Cough Syrup of Sage & Honey. It's so easy, but it's effective. Honey is more powerful than any cough medicine from drugstores. Sage is an astringent, anti-bacterial, & anti-inflammatory herb, which makes it perfect for coughs and sore throats. Sage and honey make a delicious cough syrup together, and it's simply that everyone can make one batch. It is such cough syrup that is simple and convenient. As honey is an exceptional preservative, a sample will last indefinitely.

We have listed below the ingredients that you would require for preparing this Native American herbal recipe:

- One cup or two of sage leaves, organic and fresh
- One cup or extra of honey (raw), local preferred

- One clean glass container or jar which can be tightly sealed & can contain at least twelve ounces

Given below are the detailed instructions for preparing this Native American herbal recipe. You need to follow these instructions in the given order.

- Wash & dry the sage properly.
- The leaves should be trimmed from the stems.
- Put sage leaves into the glass jar. Then pour honey over the sage leaves. It would take some while for honey to move between the leave and soak them thoroughly.
- Take a spoon and mix properly. Mix it daily. Allow it to sit for a week.
- Pull out the leaves and squeeze to take out all honey. You can also decant or leave it here & spoon it out as required into a container.
- Administer medicinally for painful throats& coughs in teaspoonfuls, or stir spoonful as a calming tea in a cup of the water (warm) with a lemon's squeeze.
- Tightly pack it and store it in the fridge. As honey is an exceptional preservative, it can last for a long time.

Native American Herbs Preparation

One of the most neglected issues when it comes to emergency preparedness is applying natural herbs and plants for medicinal use. Many people have no idea in the modern world which plants are dangerous and which plants could be used as a medicine, but it wasn't always that way. There is nothing new in using herbs and plants for medicinal use. Under the theory that man is a part of nature, Native Americans utilized them for thousands of years. Also, archaeological findings have shown that man, starting with the ancient Egyptians and Chinese has been using herbs and plants for medicinal purposes since at least 3000 BC. They used herbs and plants to cure oral disorders to stomach aches, headaches, skin rashes and more. It was not until the 1700s and 1800s that scholars and medical practitioners started to study these plants in the Western world. Today, science has progressed to the point that it is extremely rare to include natural ingredients in pharmaceutical medication, even though most of today's drugs derive from elements that exist naturally. Of course, in a survival situation, you certainly won't have any prescription meds. In this situation, the natural herbs and plants that Native Americans used hundreds of years ago would be the next best option. The few that are worth learning about are:

3.1 Blackberries

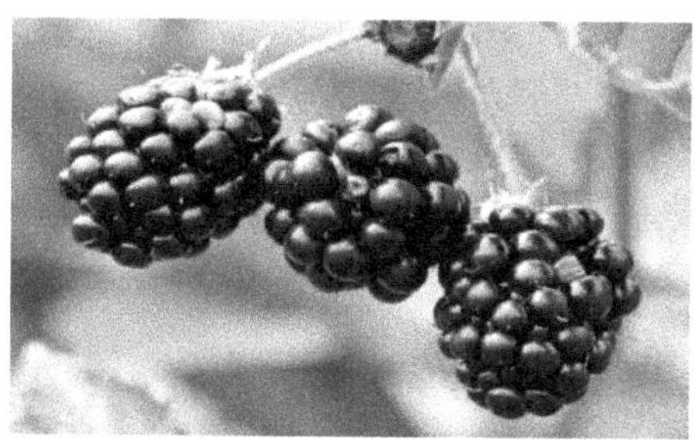

These are also the same blackberries that have healing qualities that you purchase at the store. The Cherokee tribe will use them, most importantly, to help calm stomach pain. Scientific analysis has revealed today that blackberries are high in antioxidants, which may explain why stomach pain can be minimized. Native Americans used to grind the roots and mix them with honey while consuming blackberries orally. This resulting formula would calm issues with the stomach, alleviate coughs, soothe mouth stores and provide relief to sore throats.

Wild Ginger

Wild ginger was used for medicinal purposes by many Native American tribes. The Cherokee tribe used the plant to facilitate digestion. The tribe used it to help with illnesses such as colic, intestinal bloating and gas, and aches and cramps in the stomach. To remove unnecessary mucus from the lungs, wild ginger was also used. European immigrants who settled in North America had to live without many of the Old Country's comforts of home. However, they discovered a replacement in the rhizomes of an unrelated plant that they called wild or Indian ginger in the case of ginger root (Zingiber officinale) (Asarum canadense). A member of the birthwort family is wild ginger. Around 70 species of low-growing, stem-less perennial herbs with aromatic rhizomes constitute the genus Asarum, mostly native to warm temperate eastern Asia, just a few to North America, and one to Europe.

Uses

Native Americans prepared wild ginger rhizome decoctions and infusions to deal with problems related to menstruation cycles and control irregular heartbeats. To reduce earache, Meskwaki steeped crushed rhizomes and poured the solvent into the ear. There was little denying that early European explorers learned many medical applications from Native Americans. Perhaps an Indian cure was also their teeth powder made from the pulverized bark of black alder, bayberry, and black oak combined with the powdered wild ginger rhizome. However, their use of the candied rhizome and syrup to alleviate flatulence and stomach cramps presumably resulted from similar ginger root use. The "doctrine of signatures" was another Old World influence, according to which the kidney-shaped leaves of wild ginger were a symbol that the plant was intended to be used for curing kidney disorders. Other wild ginger folk uses involved relieving fevers by triggering sweating and curing snakebite (hence one name for it, Canada snakeroot).

3.2 Buckbrush

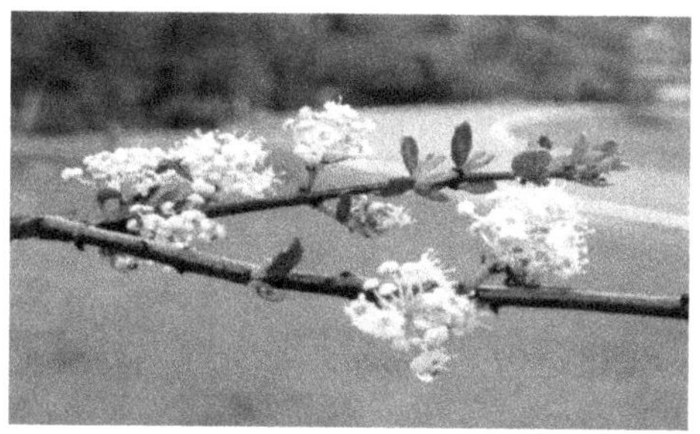

To survive, you need at least one of your kidneys to work properly, and buckbrush is one of the best natural materials to achieve your kidneys good functioning. To treat tumors and cysts, inflammation and sore throats, buckbrush can also be used. This herb was historically used with diuretic properties as a medicinal substance. It has historically been used to promote the efficient functioning of the kidneys. To treat mouth and throat problems, inflammation, and cysts and tumors, members of almost the same plant family have also been utilized.

These herbs also address particular health conditions, such as inflamed tonsils, aftercare for miscarriage, hemorrhoids, enlarged spleens and swollen lymph nodes. Its easiest and most effective use is in the form of tea. Boil some water for five to ten minutes and put the roots in it. To receive the full benefits, you may then continue to drink the resulting buckbrush tea.

3.3 Wild Black Cherry, One of the Great North American Herbs

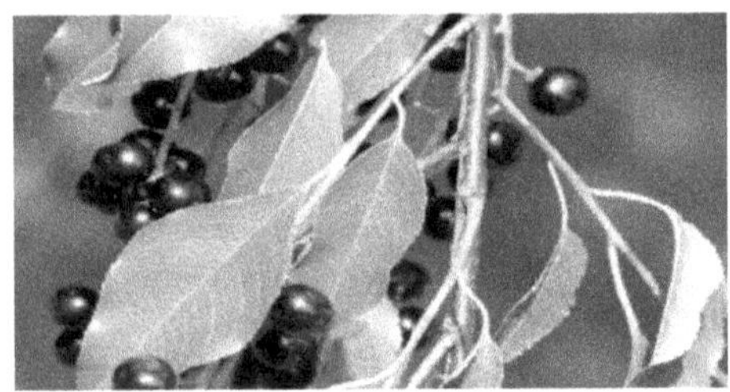

After the logging, wildfires, & other distressed soils like the yard & forest edges, these common trees pop up. They grow rapidly and are vulnerable to the disease, so you're better off learning how to recognize them than humanize them. The Prune trees upto 1 inch in diameter or, for medicine, cut down an entire young tree, scrape off bark& chop up tiny twigs. Then Wait till after the flowering & dry properly before using it in remedies. For acidic, aggravated, spastic coughs & chest symptoms, like wood smoke & wildfires, cherry bark is outstanding. This calms spasms & allows the lungs to open. It acts well as dried plant tincture (to balance bark tannins, add 10 percent glycerine), tea (that is best in tepid or is not relatively boiling water), otherwise processed cold honey or syrups. Often known as chokecherry, wild cherry bark (Prunus serotina, P. virginiana) is one of many herbal remedies containing amygdalin, also known as prunasin, a toxic glycoside contained in seeds of several species of Rosaceae, including peaches, bitter almonds, apricots and loquat, a herb used to alleviate coughing in traditional Chinese medicine (TCM). It is found in blackberry leaves as well. Prunasin's unique property is its ability to prevent the cough reflex, especially in the case of dry cough, which has become one of the most severe long-term complications following influenza in recent years. One of the most successful therapies for asthma, bronchitis and whooping cough that has spread through the US's sectors in recent months is a tea of wild cherry bark and coltsfoot.

Uses

Although herbalists promote the use of wild cherry bark as a sovereign cure for coughs in tea and alcoholic tincture extracts, a misunderstanding occurs when writers describing edible plants are likely to highlight the possible toxic properties of wild cherry. Thus, this flower, in particular arrives with significant mixed messages for the herbalist and user to wade through. There is a scenario in which the adage "the poison is in the dose" remains true. It is possible to safely use wild cherry inner bark.

Historical and Modern Use of Wild Cherry

Native American settlers first learned the medicinal uses of wild cherry bark throughout the United States. In reality, Meriwether Lewis was treated with a twig tea of wild cherry bark on his famous expedition for a severe gastrointestinal illness. Its uses as a general GI tonic, a remedy for diarrhea and sore throat, coughs and colds, as a purgative and applied topically to avoid bleeding, native individuals are on record. Many cautions about its use for pregnant mothers and children under two years of age. Nevertheless, Native Americans employed wild cherry to ease labor pains and gave it to nursing mothers who "drank the tea to pass on the medicinal effects to their infants." From 1820 to 1970, wild cherry bark was mentioned as an official in the US Pharmacopeia, arguably a more enlightened time before Big Pharma systematically established itself. To facilitate rapid recovery, herbalists typically prescribe heroic doses of herbs, especially in acute circumstances. An exception will be this herb. The tea is usually prepared by steeping two tsps of wild cherry bark in one cup of boiling water for ten minutes; it will be safe to drink roughly 3 cups every day. It will also be perfect for anywhere from thirty to sixty drops three times every day of the tincture. Besides being a cough inhibitor, wild cherry bark has numerous other applications. It is used to avoid bleeding, diarrhea and hemorrhoids, for sore throats, colds, and as an astringent. It can also be used to treat jaundice and as a digestive stimulant. The same properties that relax dry, irritable coughs are also useful for anxious palpitations, such that wild cherry bark serves the circulatory and nervous systems as a moderate sedative and other mucosal surfaces, including those of the gastrointestinal and urinary tracts. Bark tea fomentations may be used externally to alleviate pain and facilitate the curing of injury and burn caused by inflammation. Herbalists also recommend an ointment as a remedy for hemorrhoids and wounds.

Last but not least, as an eyewash for inflamed skin, the wild cherry bark's anti-inflammatory properties are especially effective. Wild cherry bark has been commonly used in formula for people of all ages, often in tea or syrup for cough and upper respiratory disease, for more than 30 years. People with asthma and chronic emphysema can make tea from a handful of equivalent portions of the following dried herbs simmered in a quart of water for 20 minutes:

- Wild cherry bark
- A quarter part lobelia herb

- Several slices of raw ginger
- Coltsfoot
- Comfrey root
- Elecampane
- Yerba santa

Effective preparation

Wild cherry bark is safe and very powerful. Double water percolation is a common and effective cherry bark syrup preparation. In a second cone filled with good old-fashioned sugar, the first percolation drips water through the cone (use organic if it makes you feel better). You are left with a sweet almond tasting syrup by the time it stops pouring, which masks the bitterness of the cherry bark. It may be used for children and adults as a respiratory antispasmodic and anti-tussive, expectorant, and to relieve throat pain. It has served well with pertussis, a tickle in the throat, dry hacking coughs, chest tension, and moderate wheezing that accompanies a respiratory infection.

Marshmallow Leaf and Root

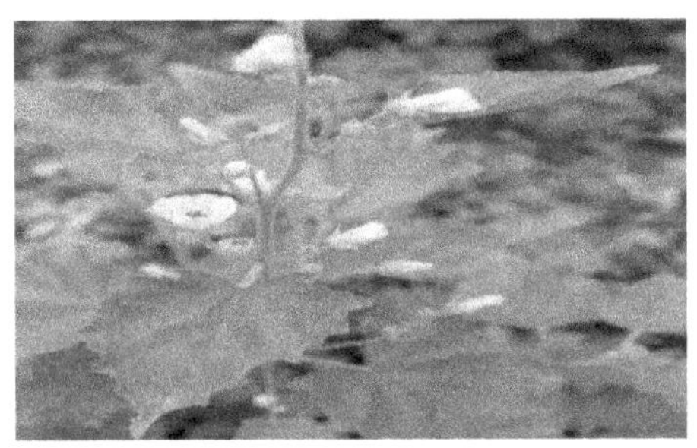

Whenever the lungs and respiratory system are dry or irritated, mallows are the ultimate moisturizing herbs as they are calming & slimy & useful. Meadow environment or the garden pampered beds with lush, mildly moist soil & partial or full sun are the right growth conditions for Mallows. In a variety of habitats, wild mallows flourish. Once you discover its happy spot, it is easy to cultivate; it should be harvested earlier in the season before the descent of Japan's hungry beetles. The marshmallow root produces the most important slime. They are in abundance, and leaves are not difficult to harvest. Feel free to get the flowers included. The calming mucilage contains the finest water extracts: cold infusions, syrup, tea, broth. The taste is moderate and mildly sweet, and more herbal & drying the herbs are excellent in recipes. Avoid the alcohol, except maybe for preservation in limited amounts.

It is possible to showcase its ability to support the respiratory system, which happens to be amongst the biggest properties of Marshmallow Root. It is an outstanding anti-inflammatory as well. This herbaceous perennial plant belongs to the family of mallows. While it belongs to the same genus as the hollyhocks, it appears to be much larger. All have observed the delicate and hairy leaves at least once. Its flowers are white and red with a very thick root. These roots are potent because they produce massive quantities of mucilage. If you want to keep it, you can use its flowers, leaves and stems, which have the same properties as the root. It is beneficial for treating bronchitis, cough, and it is ideal for relieving toothache and mouth sores. Native Americans used this plant to treat wounds and snakebites.

Natural Benefits

For an incredibly long time, herbal remedies have been around. Years before western medicine was around, predecessors of all civilizations used herbal medicines. Few herbals, including marshmallow root, have just as many values, advantages, and medical uses. This is a herbal remedy that is safe and perfect. For example, it may be used as a balm and a digestive aid because of its therapeutic feature. Plus, it can assist with breathing and skin conditions by applying it externally. Using the marshmallow balm for cough and mucus is the normal approach. This will soften the alveoli as soon as you try it, and you will feel a lot better. It is not to mention that expelling mucus and coping with asthma and bronchitis is a wonderful support function of this herb. It is the best combination for treating cystitis and other urinary tract disorders if you blend a marshmallow infused with corn silk. Swallowing this plant will help you enhance renal transit rapidly and ease any existing tension in the kidneys. It is beneficial to apply marshmallow as a poultice for all sorts of skin conditions to treat burns and bad wounds. Plus, in a rich infusion, marshmallow flowers will help you minimize inflammation. Only make sure that you apply it to the affected area. It's almost hard to beat its multiple therapeutic properties; you can't argue it's a one-of-a-kind treat.

- Splendid for treating respiratory illness
- Gives excellent results for urinary tract issues
- Handy first aid for burns and wounds

Revolutionary American Manufacturing

Americans are among the world's biggest customers today. They purchase about 90 million pounds a year of this herb in different forms. These snacks were developed by mixing sugar, egg whites and mallow root sap before modern manufacturing. This has now been largely replaced by corn syrup, starch, gelatin and water. It is useful for lowering the sugar index for people with diabetes before all sugar ingredients are added to the marshmallow root.

Plantain Leaf

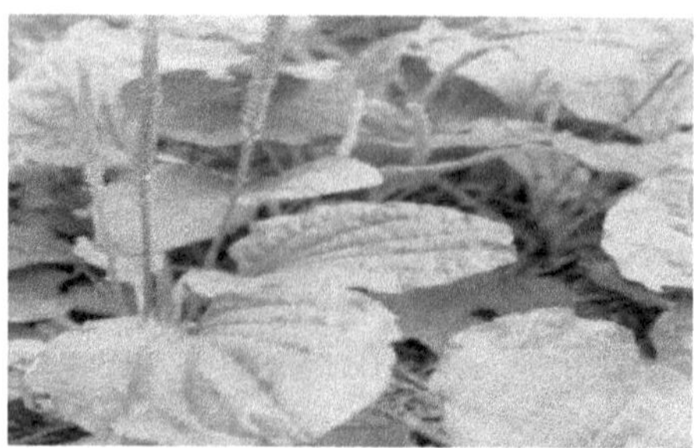

In lawns, roads, and perturbed soils, this popular weed can be found. The healthier the soil, the larger it becomes. Plantain is most famously used for insect bites and bee stings as a poultice, but the leaves are also calming and curing when used in lung recipes. In addition to boggy dampness, they relieve irritation and dryness, softly moisturizing while still serving to clean, tighten, and tone the mucus covering. They could also provide antimicrobial activity. Consider this for syrups and tea. It has a moderate, friendly and lightly tannic flavor.

What is Plantain?

A common backyard herb with large leaves is Plantain or Plantago Major. Many people, while it is an extremely useful herb, think of it as a weed. Legend has it found by Alexander the Great and carried back to Europe with him in 327 BCE. It has been referred to by Native Americans as the Whiteman's Foot, as everywhere they go, it appeared to pop up, and it's seen as an invasive, noxious weed in some areas. However, it is a useful little herb. Many civilizations worldwide also used it, and the Saxons considered it one of their nine holy herbs. It was considered an early Christian sign of the faithful's path and is referred to as an aphrodisiac by many cultures today. These leaves are very edible and are sometimes used raw & cooked as greens. The Older leaves also have a better taste, often objectionable, and can be tough and stringy, but can be used for tea making. Plantain has a very high concentration of vitamins C and A and calcium. Native Americans used plantain leaves medicinally to ease the bee stings & bites of insects, avoid the itching caused by poison ivy& more allergic rashes, & facilitate healing of sores& bruises. Plantain tea could even be used as an expectorant and mouthwash to help cure and avoid sores in the mouth. Most recently, plantain has been promoted to avoid smoking, bringing another application to the versatile herb's useful applications. Plantain was used in some cultures of Native Americans as a panacea and for some very great reasons. Also, being antitoxic and anti-inflammatory, many of its active components possess antibacterial and antimicrobial effects. A common remedy for bug & animal bites is the leaves, which can be chewed or shredded. The antibacterial activity helps deter infection & anti-inflammatory helps relieve discomfort, burning & itching. To study the effects on reducing blood sugar, some research is underway.

The Many Uses of Plantain

Plantain leaf can be made into a tea, tincture or infusion. Plantain leaf can also be used internally:

- To help get Cholesterol to healthy Levels
- For Hemorrhoid relief
- To help get relief from Irritable Bowel Syndrome
- To help calm the bowels during Constipation or Diarrhea
- To aid people suffering from Diabetes
- To treat kidney and bladder problems.
- To aid with a Bladder infection, ITIs and similar problems.
- It is safe for children
- It can be used for treating indigestion and ulcers

Plantain Leaf is also very soothing on external inflammation:

- Bites
- Burns
- Cuts
- Yeast
- Stings
- Rashes
- Eczema
- Psoriasis
- Varicose Veins

How to Use Plantain

If your yard grows fresh plantain, you should make sure it has not been sprayed with chemicals or pets and use it in teas or salads with young leaves. Make a poultice of fresh plantain leaf or bentonite clay with water to form a paste for stings and bites. When applied to the bite or sting, it will quickly take away the discomfort. Chew up a plantain leaf and spit on the bite if you don't have the other ingredients close by. It sounds disgusting, but it relieves the pain tremendously. An injection of strong tea of plantain leaf (dried or fresh) would cool the burn and ease the discomfort when sprayed on a sunburn. This can also aid Poison Ivy rashes and reactions. It would help if you steeped plantain leaves (fresh or dried) in apple cider vinegar for a couple of weeks to produce an even better solution and then strain. The flavored vinegar can very easily alleviate swelling, burning, and skin pain. Indigestion, heartburn or IBS can be soothed with a cup of plantain tea from fresh or dried leaves. It is a source of relief for all sorts of digestive problems. It also helps in treating UTIs, urinary infections or kidney infections.

White Pine

The eastern white pine is a native of North America, growing from Newfoundland to Manitoba and eastern Canada. The resin and needles were believed to have medicinal value by the First Nations. As a soothing ointment, the resin, which has certain antiseptic qualities, was smeared on wounds and boiled up to produce a tonic drink. Rich in vitamin C, the needles provided a tea that helped prevent and cure scurvy. Pine was a common ingredient in many mixtures during the heyday of patent medicines in the late 1800s. Pine has good selling potential and possesses certain antiseptic properties: the strong smell reached blocked sinuses and indicated that a strong remedy must be at work. Beyond the apparent one of providing wood, Eastern white pine also had many non-medicinal applications. First Nations used the resin to seal the seams in canoes; pine resins eventually became the basis of consumer goods like pitch and turpentine. The eastern white pine is mainly harvested for its lumber and pulp. The oils used for medicinal purposes are a by-product.

Worldwide, there are over one hundred species of pine, and most have medicinal uses. The needles, inner bark, and resin have been used by civilizations worldwide for similar ailments. Internally, for coughs, colds, asthma, and urinary tract and sinus diseases, pine is a typical treatment. Topically, pine is used in arthritic disorders to combat skin diseases and to lessen joint inflammation. About twenty species of pine have been used in a similar medicinal manner by native communities throughout the continent, including the Chippewa, Cherokee, Iroquois, Apache, Hopi and numerous other groups.

Medicinal Use of Pine Needles

The fresh needles and buds collected in the springtime are called "pine tops." They are boiled in water, and for fevers, coughs, and colds, the tea is consumed. The needles are also used for their diuretic features, helping to improve urination. Pine-top tea, particularly given the abundance of pines in the area, is one of the most valuable historical medicines of the rural south-eastern United States. Famed Alabama herbalist Tommie Bass uses the needles in a steam inhalation to break up the lungs' tenacious phlegm.

For this reason, you may mix pine tops with sprigs of fresh thyme and bee balm. Pine induces relaxation by its relaxing expectorant, antimicrobial, & anti-inflammatory characteristics in sinus and lung congestion. Vitamin C is also in the fresh, younger needles. Try mixing peppermint and catnip as a tea with pine needles, which can be sipped to soothe cold symptoms during the day. For the entire household, this mixture is a healthy cure.

- Mighty Pine Tea
- 1-quart water
- A fistful of pine needle tops (about five to seven branch tips; fresh or dried)
- One and a half tbsp dried peppermint
- One tbsp dried catnip

For twenty minutes, boil the pine needle tops in water. Turn the heat off, and the peppermint and catnip are inserted. Cover and allow to steep for an extra twenty minutes. If needed, strain and add honey. While hot, sip on the tea, reheating each cup during the day as needed. Adults can consume three cups a day. The dosages for children should be lowered proportionally.

Pine Bark

The inner bark contains more resin than the needles and is more astringent. It has traditionally been used for muscular aches and pains as an antimicrobial wash and poultice and infused into bathwater. It is sometimes boiled in water and consumed for coughs and colds as a cure. The knotty pine wood of many pine types is mixed into wine in Traditional Chinese Medicine and then used topically for joint pain.

Pine Resin

There are numerous local first-aid applications of the resin, also called pitch. It is used as an antimicrobial dressing for wounds and to extract splinters. Pine resin has been used internally as a strong expectorant in minute quantities. You can use pine pitch to pull out splinters, glass, and the contaminants left from toxic bug bites prepared as a salve. Pine resin salve is effective in reducing muscle aches and inflammation of the joints.

Pine Pitch Band-Aids: Forest First-Aid

Take a semi-hard but pliable piece of pitch and form it over the affected region into a flat bandage. While also being anti-inflammatory and antimicrobial, this basic first-aid has excellent drawing ability. Cover it and leave it on overnight with a Band-Aid or clean bandage.

- Pine Pitch Salve
- One part clean pine pitch
- Two parts extra-virgin olive oil
- Grated beeswax beads

Melt the olive oil pitch using a double boiler (1 part pitch to 2 parts olive oil, by volume) until it is completely melted (it's okay if a little resin stays solid). Add the grated beeswax (one-part beeswax per four parts of the combined pitch and liquid oil). Before inserting lids, pour into jars and leave to cool.

Safety & Contraindications

In pregnancy, should not use pine needles and prevent the long-term internal use of bark. With long-term use of heavy doses or with sensitive individuals, the pine needles and pine bark may cause kidney irritation. But in minute doses under the supervision of a certified herbalist, you can use pine resin internally. You should be confident that you have identified pine correctly, and it's not a look-alike or a sound-alike.

Tobacco

There are more than 60 species of tobacco, officially called Nicotiana, that are mostly indigenous to Australia and America. For social, religious, ceremonial purposes and medicinal remedies, plants had also assumed greater importance in Native American culture. Leaves have long been used to remedy boils, poison, skin conditions, measles, vertigo, and to cure mosquitoes and snakebites to prevent nausea, colic, worms, kidney problems, fever, colic, convulsions, toothache. Tobacco and other plant mixtures are grown or harvested and used for ceremonial or medicinal purposes by American Indians, and Alaska Natives are traditional tobacco. For centuries, traditional tobacco has been used as a medicine with cultural and theological significance by American Indian nations. Many tribes preserve the teachings and legends about the roots of tobacco. These teachings deal with tobacco in its simplest form, known today as the Nicotiana rustica tobacco plant, and can contain other indigenous plants' mixtures. The traditional preparation and use of tobacco differ across tribes and territories, with traditional tobacco not widely used by Alaskan natives. These variations are due to the many distinct teachings of the North American Tribes. The functions of cultivating, processing, and preparing conventional tobacco in certain communities are held by unique classes of individuals who use traditional methods to prepare tobacco for a particular use. The significance of maintaining a positive attitude and thoughts even when working with traditional tobacco is one common teaching. Traditional tobacco is a medicine that may be used to promote emotional, physical, spiritual and community well-being in a prescribed manner. A traditional tobacco gift is a sign of respect and might even be offered when requesting assistance, guidance, or protection. In herbal medicine, traditional tobacco is often used specifically for curing. It can be burnt or smoked in a pip, but the smoke is normally not inhaled. The smoke from burning tobacco has the function of bringing thoughts and prayers to the divine world or the Creator in certain teachings. Traditional tobacco is not linked with tolerance and adverse health effects when used properly. In the planning and usage of conventional tobacco, the care and reverence involved are part of centuries of practice that ties today's children, adults, and elders with those who existed years ago. Today and for future years to come, continued use of traditional tobacco promotes a decent life and a healthy society.

3.4 Cattail

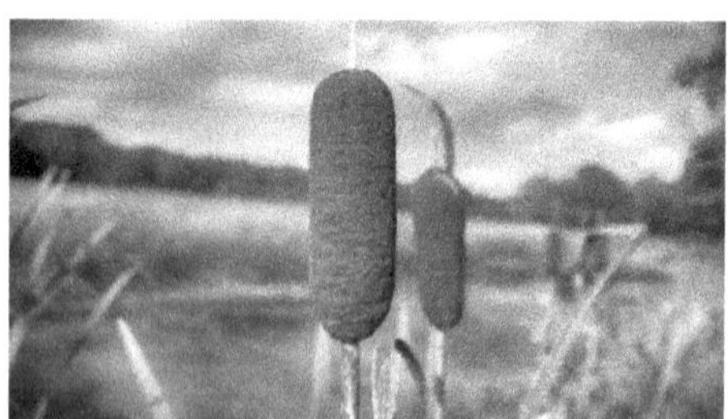

Cattail is more like a prevention therapy than an active drug. Except for the seeds and the leaves, any part of the plant can be consumed. For open wounds such as bruises, abrasions, and scrapes, Cattail is best used as an antiseptic. The Cattail's root may be simply broken open and brought into close contact with the open wound, then tied with a rope or paracord. Also, for this same therapeutic purpose, cattail ash may be used.

Simply put it into close contact with the wound that is open. Currently, the legend says that, with a little support from the humble Cattail, the US was on the brink of winning World War 2. More edible starch than almost any other green plant is produced by Cattail (starch per acre). From this point of view, rice, potatoes, yams, or taros are less nutritious than Cattail. Lichen is the only plant capable of beating cattails in terms of carbs per acre (starch is the essential carbohydrate), although this is not a green plant. An acre of cattails can, however, yield 6.5K pounds of flour annually on average.

Health benefits of Cattail

Cattail is one of the plants that are cultivated worldwide that are good and nutrient-rich. Some of the common health benefits of cattail consumption are described in detail below:

Improves digestion

Cattail consists of a good amount of soluble and insoluble fiber necessary for the digestive system's proper functioning. Soluble fibers counter cholesterol accumulation and insoluble fiber enables waste to pass out of the environment. This adds to lower chances of hemorrhoids or even constipation. So use cattail in your diet to eliminate all of the issues associated with digestion.

Calorie rich

If you are undernourished and want to add some weight, the easiest way is to pair Cattails' rich diet with a wholesome dinner. The weight gain process is facilitated because the cattail is high in nutrients and calories. It is also one of the beneficial choices for underweight individuals to achieve the required body weight.

Skin Health

Cattail consists of immense quantities of nutrients and organic compounds, which primarily promotes its ability to cure boils, sores, lessen the occurrence of scars, and add to its effect on the skin. Topically, cattail jelly should be used for mosquito bites, but the flour also has an anti-inflammatory ability that reduces some affected discomfort and severity.

Hypertension

Adrenal glands are given sufficient assistance to minimize stress levels due to Cattail's protein and carbohydrate content. It tends to increase the rate of metabolism and hence lowers stress.

Diabetes

Phytochemicals are needed for insulin absorption. Your system can combat diabetes mellitus, which is non-insulin-dependent, by taking Cattail daily. So eating Cattail daily to fight diabetes is fruitful.

Cancer Prevention

However, this field of study is somewhat new and somewhat contentious, but research is underway on cattails' potential to prevent cancer. Chinese researchers are leading a promising new field of study, but its antioxidant effects on cancer cells are promising.

Atherosclerosis

Because of the presence of vitamin C, carotenoids and bioflavonoids, the intake of Cattail decreases LDL. These components ensure that coronary disease complications are minimized, and the LDL is cleaned out of the system. Apart from that, the absorption of cholesterol is also decreased. This suggests a lowered chance of developing atherosclerosis.

Cardio tonic and lipid-lowering effects

There is a certain composition of compounds in the Cattail, which reduces the lipids in the body and dilates the coronary artery. It is used to treat coronary conditions such as angina, hyperlipidemia, etc. It is also used for dissolving stasis. It tends to decrease lipid accumulation on the artery walls. Hence, the occurrence of heart failure is reduced.

Antiseptic Application

Cattail is famous because of its natural antiseptic quality, which has come in handy for various cultures for centuries. In wounds and other parts of the body where foreign agents, bacteria, or microbes could harm our system, the jelly-like compounds you will find between young leaves are used. This same jelly is regarded as a potent analgesic from the cattail plant, which can be eaten or applied topically to alleviate discomfort and inflammation.

Steady increase in energy

As we all know, a rich source of energy is carbohydrates. There is a decent amount of starch content in Cattail. It means that it has the potential to give you higher energy levels and even replenish energy levels from time to time if they are insufficient. The breakdown is very slow because Cattail is made up of complex carbohydrates, which means you will have all the energy you need for the day.

Slow Bleeding

Different portions of the Cattail have coagulant properties, which ensures they slow down blood supply and prevent anemia. If you are injured, this can be effective, but also if you suffer from excessive menstrual bleeding, reducing the severity. But for patients who still have moderately poor circulation, it is potentially harmful because it essentially slows blood down while also stimulating the skin's coagulant response.

How to Eat

- Several parts of the herb, including dormant sprouts on the leaves' roots and bases, ripe pollen, the stem and starchy roots, are edible.
- Raw or cooked roots are edible.
- They can be boiled and eaten similar to potatoes or macerated to create sweet syrup and then boiled.
- Roots may also be dried or ground into a powder and subsequently used or added to cereal flours as a thickener in soups, etc., and this protein-rich powder is used to produce cookies, etc.

Young shoots are eaten raw or cooked during the spring.

The base of the mature stem can also be consumed both raw or cooked.

It is often edible raw, fried or prepared in a soup, the tender, young flowering stem.

Pollen is edible, raw, cooked or refined into a rich in protein additive used in the processing of bread, porridge, etc.

Tiny seeds can be roasted or fried, and edible oil can be extracted from the seeds.

3.5 Dandelion

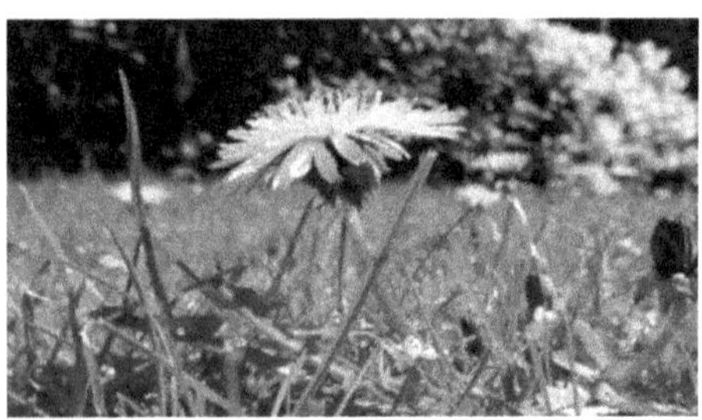

We should all be acquainted with what dandelions are, and the first to find out how to use them medically were the Native Americans. Did you know, for instance, that eating a dandelion salad (where you eat the leaves) will help relieve a sore throat? Do you also know the dandelion is a diuretic and can help you pass urine as a result? What you'll have to do is have some dandelion tea.

Smilax Bona-Nox

This herb has been used as a mild diuretic and a blood purifier. Used in the form of tea, this herb, using its roots, has also been used to cure arthritis. It can also help heal mild wounds, bruises, scrapes, and sores; the plant's leaves and bark should be mixed with lard. Sarsaparilla is from the genus Smilax, a tropical herb. The growing, woody vine grows deep inside the rainforest canopy. It is native to South America, Jamaica, Mexico, Honduras, the Caribbean, and the West Indies.

Sarsaparilla drink

The common name of a soft drink popular in the early 1800s is also Sarsaparilla. As a home cure, the drink was used and was also served in bars. The sarsaparilla soft drink was normally made from another plant called sassafras, contrary to common opinion. It has been identified as being similar to root beer or birch beer in flavor. In some Southeast Asian countries, the drink is still popular but is no longer common in the US.

The benefits

Sarsaparilla produces a wealth of compounds from plants known to have a therapeutic impact on the human body. Chemicals such as saponins can help relieve pain in the joints and itching of the skin and kill bacteria. Other chemicals may be useful to minimize inflammation and to protect the liver from damage. It is important to remember that human experiments are either very old or absent from these claims.

Psoriasis

Decades earlier, the advantages of sarsaparilla root for treating psoriasis were recorded. One research showed that in persons with psoriasis, sarsaparilla healed skin lesions significantly. The researchers proposed that one of the key steroids of sarsaparilla, called sarsaponin, can bind to and extract from the body the endotoxins liable for the lesions in psoriasis patients.

Arthritis

A potent anti-inflammatory, Sarsaparilla is. This aspect also helps treat inflammatory disorders such as rheumatoid arthritis and other triggers of joint pain and gout-induced swelling.

Syphilis

Against toxic bacteria and other microorganisms that have infiltrated the body, Sarsaparilla has shown activity. It has been used for decades to cure major diseases such as leprosy and syphilis, but it does not work and present-day antibiotics and antifungals. Syphilis is a disease of sexual transmission caused by a bacterium. Another debilitating illness caused by bacteria is leprosy. In recent studies, the antimicrobial role of Sarsaparilla has been reported. One paper looked at the behavior of over 60 different sarsaparilla-isolated phenolic compounds. These compounds were tested by researchers against six kinds of bacteria and one fungus. The researchers reported 18 compounds having antimicrobial activity against the bacteria and one against the fungus, respectively.

Cancer

Recent research has shown that sarsaparilla has anti-cancer effects in multi-cancer cell lines in mice. Preclinical trials have also demonstrated the anti-tumor effects of sarsaparilla in breast cancer tumors and liver cancer. To discover that if sarsaparilla could be used in cancer prevention and care, further research is needed.

Protecting the liver

Sarsaparilla also showed beneficial effects on the liver. A study performed in liver-damaged rats showed that compounds abundant in sarsaparilla flavonoids could reverse liver damage and make it function at its best.

How to Eat

- The roots can be added to soups and stews.
- The young shoots can be consumed raw. They can also be cooked like asparagus.
- The berries can be consumed raw. They can also be cooked.
- The tendrils can also be consumed.
- It is generally used as an ingredient in soft drinks.

Curly Dock

Used as an ingredient in salads, curly dock is filled with good vitamins and minerals and has a sweet yet sour flavor. It is also a rich source of iron. It was often thought that the herb had laxative effects. The Cherokee mixed it with beeswax, a little oil, and ground it up. The salve has been used with mild burns, sores, rashes and other skin irritations as an ointment. Due to their tart, lemony taste, widespread availability, and the fact that they were free for the taking, docks were common wild edibles during the Great Depression. Today, this popular and tasty edible weed has been overlooked by most people. Docks are annual plants emerging from taproots, and they are most commonly found in open fields and along roadsides in neglected, disturbed soil.

Which Docks Are Edible?

There are several edible docks, but the most popular in the USA and Europe are curly docks and broad-leaved docks. Other docks that are edible have R. (Western dock) occidentalis, R. (yard dock) longifolius, and R. Stenphyllus stenphylus (field dock). R. In the American Southwest, hymenosepalus (wild rhubarb) is widespread in the desert. It is bigger than many other docks and is more succulent. For many Native American tribes, it has been a common source of food and dye.

Parts used for food

stems,Young leaves, seed.

Food uses of dock

They've tart, leaves tasting like lemon & are used in cooking similarly. Most young plants are always the finest to make a delicious 'spinach' while some find the flavor 'sour' yet 'hearty.' Use bacon, butter, eggs (hard-boiled) & seasoning to serve the greens. Like the vine leaves and rice, cheese filling and herb, the leaves may also be stuffed. Dried, they may be used for potatoes, rice, fish, or the sandwich spread as a seasoning. They produce vast amounts of fruits & nuts that can also be boiled into ground or mush to make bread, muffins and gravies & added to meal or flour. As a replacement for rhubarb pie, the young plants' stems could be sliced, simmered & sweetened with honey.

Nutritional profile of dock

The plants are also very nutritious. For instance, Curly Dock has far extra vitamin C compared to oranges and much extra vitamin A compared to carrots. This also contains B2 and B1vitamins& iron.

Dock recipes

Rice, Dock, seaweed parcelsand feta Cheese

Herbal medicine uses of dock

To soothe nettle stings, leaves are excellently used and sometimes grow near the offending plant. Calming properties were used for scalds, blisters and sprains, and have also been used for soothing stings and insect bites. They were a common treatment for staunching bleedings or blood purification. To cure wounds, the juice from leaves may be put in as a rub. The seeds were used to cure liver disorders, jaundice, skin conditions, constipation, boils, rheumatism, and diarrhea. The roots were used to cure coughs, colds and bronchitis.

3.6 Elderflower

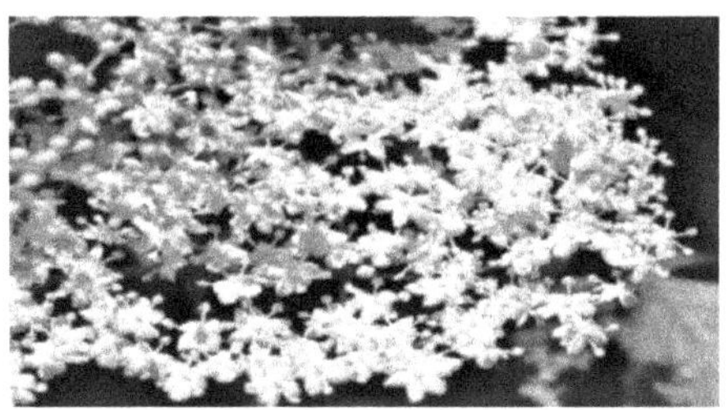

In various ways, elderflower can be consumed: some of the most common are jelly, syrup, and tea. But be careful, for the flower section itself is the only edible component. Since they are poisonous, the leaves, roots, twigs and stems cannot be eaten safely.

What's used for medicinal purposes is the extract of the elderflower. The extract should, precisely, be used as a remedy for:Sweating

- Influenza
- The Common Cold
- Bleeding
- Bronchitis
- Constipation

- Colds

3.6 Flaxseed

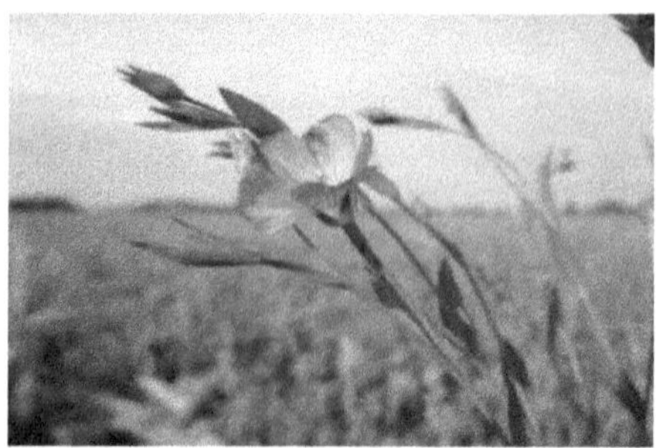

To help heal the kidney, flaxseed has been used. It can also be used to relieve heart-related complications and sore throats. .As long as you don't eat it while it's raw or unripe, flaxseed can also be eaten in whatever way you see fit. The recommended way to use it is when it is in powdered form or dried form.

3.7 Lavender

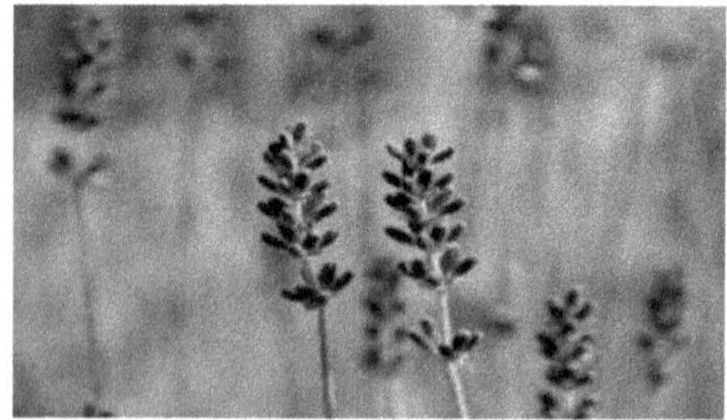

Lavender could be the treatment you are searching for if you have suffered from any sleep-related issues. During a survival scenario, having plenty of sleep would be crucial to keep the energy levels up. To find it easy to sleep and calm the discomfort from headaches, the Native Americans will use the scent of lavender. It is extremely easy to make lavender oil. Steep the branches in olive oil (or water if you're in a condition of survival), and you'll be set.

3.7 Mint

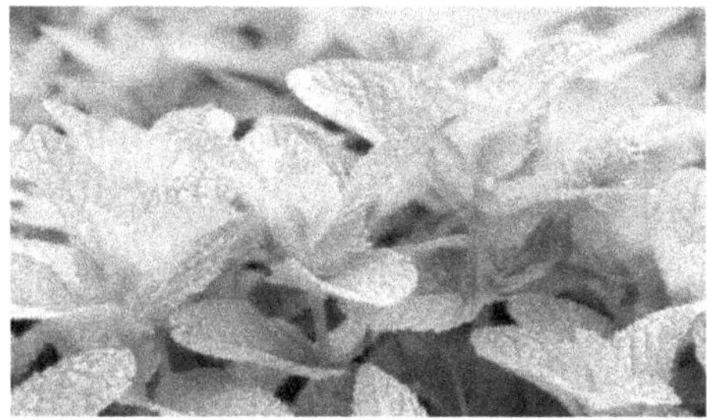

Mint is well-known, even to those unfamiliar with herbal medicines. Besides being rich in magnesium, calcium, phosphate, and potassium, mint is safe because it is very high in Vitamin A and Vitamin C. To lower blood pressure and alleviate discomfort in the digestive tract, the Cherokee tribe will make mint tea. Crush the mint leaves to cure itchy spots and skin rashes, mix them with a little water to make an ointment and then rub the mixture directly to the infected region.

Mullein

For lung and respiratory issues, this traditional herb may help. The Cherokee burnt the mullein roots, inhaled the smoke they felt, opened the airways and relieved the mucous membrane's inflammation that lines the respiratory tract. For curing joint pain and migraine headaches, the flowers may be used to prepare a sedative drink. For asthma, whooping cough, measles, bronchitis, hoarseness, asthma, earaches, colds, chills, flu, swine flu, fever, nausea, sore throat, and tonsillitis, Mullein is used. Asthma, diarrhea, colic, stomach bleeding, migraines, knee pain, and gout are also found to be successfully treated with this herb. To improve urine production, it is also used as a diuretic. It is also used as a sedative. For cuts, bruises, burns, hemorrhoids, frostbite and skin infections, Mullein is applied to the skin (cellulitis). To soften and protect the skin, the leaves are used topically. In manufacturing, Mullein is used in alcoholic drinks as a flavoring component. Mullein is a respiratory tonic that is supreme, healthy and profound. It helps to open the lungs, relieves spasms, tightness and cough, and alleviates dryness and discomfort. In the garden, this common weed may be seeded. In lawns, meadows, and gardens, Mullein prefers the sunny, open, and disturbed soil. It is a biennial of self-seeding. This can move about from year. Throughout the season, harvest the happy-looking leaves for tea, sugar, steam, or tincture, but be cautious when spotting the plant before it flowers. Mullein has a slight fragrance and flavor. Make sure to strain the irritating hair through a paper filter.

About mullein oil

Mullein oil is derived from the plant's flowers or leaves. The oil is used for earaches, eczema, and many other skin disorders as a treatment. Based on a trial of 171 children aged 5 and 18 years old with an ear infection, one study showed some benefit for ear pain. With or without a topical anesthetic, they were given herbal drops or antibiotics. Researchers have discovered that herbal drops decrease discomfort. They also emphasized that they cost less than antibiotics and had no side effects.

Mullein oil two ways

Mullein oil can be produced by either cold (passive) or hot (active) processing from either dry or fresh parts of the plant.

Hot oil infusion

This method involves softly heating a carrier oil, like olive oil, with mullein leaves and/or flowers for up to three hours using a double boiler technique. Then it strains and stores the product.

Cold-steeped oil

For 7 to 10 days, the cold process typically involves steeping dried flowers and/or leaves in a carrier oil. Mullein oil is now widely available online and at health food stores.

Benefits

Some active compounds of mullein include:

- saponins, that have pain-relieving, anti-inflammatory and antitumor properties
- flavonoids, that possess antioxidant as well as anti-inflammatory properties
- phenylethanoid glycosides, that have antioxidant, anti-inflammatory and antiviral properties
- iridoids, that possess anti-inflammatory properties

Antiviral properties

Verbascum species have been found to demonstrate antiviral activity against influenza A and herpes in several laboratory experiments. One laboratory research observed improved antiviral activity against influenza by mixing the drug amantadine with mullein. Mullein leaf is also sold in various forms:

- Tea
- Extract
- Oil

- Powder
- Capsule
- Elixir

Creams are often produced using the dried and raw forms (of the herb or flower). Some naturopathic practitioners and herbalists recommend mullein for curing inflammatory and respiratory issues, but there is not adequate clinical proof of its efficacy at present.

The takeaway

Herbal medicines can deliver real benefits, whether it is a relaxing tea or soothing balm. For thousands of years, Mullein has been around. For treating many problems, like cough and other respiratory conditions, its leaves and flowers have been used. It is available as tinctures, elixirs, tablets, and teas. With few reports of side effects, it's usually considered safe. For earaches and certain skin disorders, Mullein oil has been used.

3.8 Rosemary

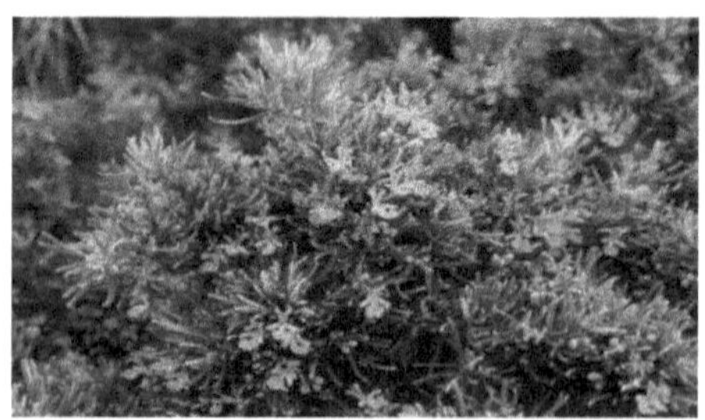

Many Native American tribes knew Rosemary to be a holy herb, and with good reason: it is simply one of the most powerful natural plants for relieving joint and muscle pain. Rosemary will also help strengthen the immune system, the nervous system, indigestion, and circulatory system. It's one of the best plants you can get your hands on.

And all you've got to do is add that to the food. Rosemary has a warm plus bitter taste, and many foods offer a nice flavor and fragrance with this plant.

Moreover, it is possible to use Rosemary in tea or as an essential oil or liquid extract. Rosemary is famous for its flavor and smell; it is also recognized for the many health benefits it provides. For decades, Rosemary has been used for medical purposes as a healthy source of calcium, iron and vitamins A, C, and B-6.

Some of Rosemary's several possible health advantages include:

- Rosemary is a great source of vitamins as well as anti-inflammatory compounds that are known to help strengthen the immune system and increase circulation in the blood.
- Rosemary is known as a cognitive stimulant that can help to enhance the efficiency and performance of memory. Alertness, intellect, and concentration are all improved significantly by its use.

In people with persistent anxiety or stress hormone imbalances, rosemary aroma has been related to improving mood, calming the mind, and alleviating stress.

It has been effective in stimulating hair growth. Moreover, rosemary oil has been known to inhibit baldness, slow graying of hair, and cure dandruff and dry scalp.

For gastrointestinal disorders, including intestinal gas, heartburn, liver and gallbladder problems, and lack of appetite, rosemary is also used.

Rosemary is especially useful against bacterial infections. It is associated with staph infection prevention.

Rosemary nutrients help protect skin cells from damage frequently caused by sunshine and free radicals. Although research on rosemary tea and eye health is incomplete, evidence suggests that your eyes can benefit from some compounds in the tea. Animal tests have shown that it can delay the development of age-related eye diseases by incorporating rosemary extract into other oral therapies (AREDs). One research investigated the addition of rosemary extract to traditional therapies such as zinc oxide and other antioxidant combinations of AREDs, finding that it helped delay (AMD), a common vision-affecting disorder. Other animals and laboratory tests show that rosmarinic acid in rosemary prevents the onset of cataracts and lowers the occurrence of cataracts.

When consumed in low doses, rosemary is safe, but it can lead to severe side effects, like vomiting, spasms, or even pulmonary edema, when eaten in extremely high doses. Before adding rosemary into your diet, please check with your doctor.

How to make rosemary tea

It is very simple and easy to make rosemary tea at home. You only require two ingredients, i.e water and rosemary to make rosemary tea:

- Bring to a boil ten ounces of water (295 ml).
- Insert one tsp of loose rosemary leaves into the hot water. Then put the leaves in a tea infuser. Allow them to steep for five to ten minutes. This all depends on how tasteful you like your tea.

- Using a mesh strainer with small holes, strain the rosemary leaves from the hot water or remove them from the tea infuser. Used rosemary leaves should be discarded.

- Pour in a cup of your rosemary tea and enjoy. A sweetener, like sugar, honey, or agave syrup, can be added if you prefer.

Many remarkable health benefits are provided by rosemary tea. Your mood and brain, and eye health can benefit from drinking the tea or even simply inhaling its aroma. The oxidative disruption that may lead to multiple chronic disorders can also be avoided. It's necessary, though, to be mindful of its possible interactions with certain drugs. Using only two ingredients, rosemary tea can comfortably be made at home, and it fits perfectly into an overall safe and nutritious diet.

3.9 Sumac

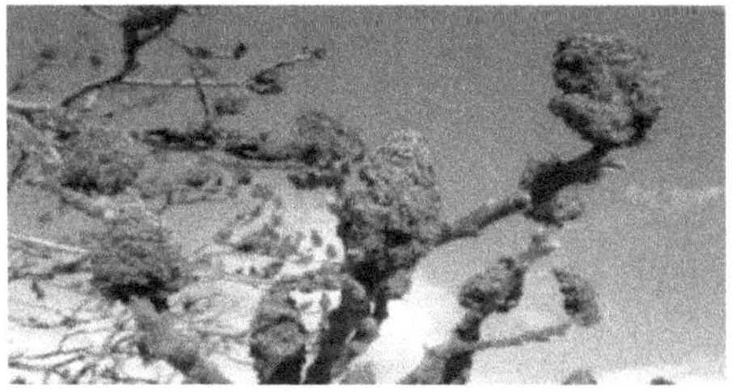

The use of Sumac excellently achieves the cure of colds, fevers, and sore throats. You'll need to make sumac tea to get these advantages. Just pick and gently crush several berry clusters, soak them overnight in a pitcher of cold water, strain the mixture to extract the berries, and enjoy it. It's so easy. The discomfort is not going to go away absolutely, but you can feel almost instant relief, and that is better than nothing. In the Middle Eastern and Mediterranean cuisines, Sumac is a common ingredient.

In comparison, in herbal therapy procedures, individuals use it therapeutically. Sumac is a flowering shrub variety that belongs to a plant family known as the Anacardiaceae. Rhus coriaria is the scientific name. Cashew & mango plants are other common members of this genus. More than two hundred separate Sumac species have been identified, all of which belong to the Rhus genus. Though Syrian Sumac or Rhus coriaria is variety people cultivate most commonly for culinary use & herbal medicine. The big, thick clusters of pea-sized, bright red fruit it provides define Sumac. People could steep fresh fruits to make tea, but they dry them & powder more often for use as a herbal substitute or the culinary seasoning.

Potential benefits

The Sumac is common known as culinary spice. The People as well usedthis in cultural practices of herbal medicine for centuries.

It is rich in important nutrients

Sumac's complete nutrient profile is largely unclear, although little research suggests that it includes a host of beneficial nutrients. These include good fats, fiber, and certain important vitamins. A 2014 study showed that roughly 71 percent carbs, 19 percent fat, & 5 percent protein constitute nutritionally dried sumac. Two distinct types of fat, called oleic acid& linoleic acid, account for the fat's bulk in sumac. The type of monounsaturated fat typically associated with cardiac health is oleic acid. It is the primary fat present in other popular foods based on plants, including avocados and olives. Linoleic acid's a kind of vital polyunsaturated fat involved in the preservation of cell membranes and healthy skin. 2004 chemical study of fresh fruit of sumac showed that fiber, a nutrient that improves digestive health, makes up over 14 percent of it. Very little information is available on the correct micronutrient contents of the sumac, although several reports indicate that this contains a trace amount of some important nutrients, at least, including the vitamins B2, B1, C, and B6.

Rich in antioxidants

Multiple antioxidant mixtures are found abundantly in Sumac. Experts agree that this could be the primary explanation for the broad medicinal potential of Sumac.

Antioxidants perform an important function to defend the cells from destruction & reduce the oxidative stress inside the body. There's also proof that antioxidants can play a role in reducing inflammation. They can help avoid inflammatory diseases, such as cancer and heart disease.

Facilitates balanced blood sugar

Some research suggests that sumac can be an important tool for treating blood sugars in people with Type 2 diabetes. A 2014 review of 41 individuals with diabetes examined the effect on blood sugar and antioxidant levels of a normal 3-gr dose of the sumac. At the end of the three-month trial, the normal blood sugar & antioxidant levels in the population consuming the sumac supplement were dramatically increased compared with those taking placebo. In another related report, forty-one people with diabetes were asked to take three grams of the sumac powder every day for three months. A 25 percent decrease in circulating the insulin was experienced by the sumac community, indicating that the insulin sensitivity might have improved substantially because of the sumac supplement.

Alleviates muscle pain

Research in 2016 gave a sumac drink or placebo to 40 healthy individuals to explore the sumac's ability to alleviate muscle pain. The group consuming sumac drinks reported substantially low exercise-based muscle pain at the end of the 4-week trial relative to the group receiving the placebo drink. Major changes in circulating the antioxidant levels were also seen in the sumac community. This might have induced the reported pain relief, the study authors proposed.

How to use

Sumac is a distinctive spice that can be used as herbal medicine or in food. Sumac is used most often by people as a seasoning. Sumac can increase the taste & color of several dishes, like many other culinary spices. It is especially common in the Middle East and Mediterranean households. Sumac has a rich red hue, a fragrance similar to citrus, and a distinct lemon juice-like tart taste. People often use it to make a sweet & sour drink called sumac lemonade. Sumac has a coarse, rough appearance when dried and ground. For many foods, namely grains, grilled meats & vegetables, baked goods, & sweets, ground sumac is excellent for adding acidity, clarity, and flavor.

Herbal supplements

As a herbal supplement, sumac is commercially available. Usually, people take this in capsule shape, but you may take this as tincture or tea as well. People dry these berries for use as a herbal remedy or culinary spice.

3.10 Yarrow

Yarrow is common worldwide and was first used by the Ancient Greeks to great effect, who used it by directly applying the leaves to stop excessive bleeding. They'd even take the yarrow juice and mix it with water as well. To better treat discomfort in the stomach or intestines, this paste would then be consumed directly. The Cherokee tribe was also well conscious of the potent medicinal properties of Yarrow, and they mainly prepared it as a tea, like the Ancient Greeks. To a cup of sugar, add a teaspoon of dried Yarrow, boil it for 10 minutes, strain the leaves and drink.

Moreover, to help cure dry skin, wrinkles, and open wounds, the Cherokee tribe would also spread Yarrow directly on the skin. Yarrow is a herb. Medicine is made with the above-ground components. Yarrow is used to curing flu, common cold, hay fever, menstrual absence, dysentery, diarrhea, lack of appetite, irritation of the gastrointestinal (GI) tract, and trigger sweating. To prevent toothaches, some people chew the fresh leaves. Yarrow is applied to the skin to stop hemorrhoid bleeding for wounds; and as a special bath for women with uncomfortable, lower vaginal, cramp-like problems.

Yarrow can be used for bloating, intestinal gas (flatulence), moderate gastrointestinal (GI) cramping, and other GI symptoms associated with other herbs. Young leaves and yarrow flowers are used in salads. As a cosmetic cleanser and in snuff, Yarrow is sometimes used in manufacturing. In shampoos, yarrow oil is used. There are several chemicals in Yarrow that could affect blood pressure and could have anti-inflammatory effects. Significant quantities of Yarrow could delay the clotting of blood.

Uses and benefits of Yarrow Tea

Yarrow tea is made from a popular medicinal herb. For thousands of years, yarrow (Achillea millefolium) has been used because of its possible health benefits. In Greek mythology, the genus name, Achillea, alludes to the warrior Achilles, when he used yarrow to heal the wounds of his soldiers. There are 140 distinct species of Achillea, with clustered flowers and hairy plus aromatic leaves. Studies suggest that, as a herbal tea, extract, or essential oil, this plant can have multiple advantages. Here are a number of the basic advantages and uses of yarrow tea.

Improves wound healing

One animal study found that there were anti-inflammatory and antioxidant properties of yarrow leaf extracts, all of which aid wound healing. In addition, this study noted that fibroblasts, the cells responsible for regenerating connective tissue and helping the body heal from damage, can be enhanced by yarrow leaf extract. Meanwhile, a 2-week study of 140 women showed that an ointment made from this herb and St. John's wort helped treat episiotomy sites, which are surgical incisions made during childbirth on the vaginal wall.

Reduces digestive issues

Yarrow has long been used to relieve intestinal conditions such as ulcers and signs of irritable bowel syndrome (IBS), including pain in the gut, diarrhea, bloating and constipation. In fact, many flavonoids and alkaloids are found in this herb, that are plant compounds known to alleviate digestive complaints. A yarrow extract tonic defended against stomach acid damage in a study in rats and exhibited anti-ulcer abilities. Another animal study showed that yarrow tea's flavonoid antioxidants can reduce inflammation, digestive spasms and other symptoms of IBS.

Alleviates symptoms of depression and anxiety

Flavonoids and alkaloids can alleviate symptoms of depression and anxiety in yarrow tea. Studies suggest that plant-based alkaloids such as those present in yarrow tea decrease corticosterone secretion, a hormone that is high during chronic stress. One research showed that essential yarrow oils given orally to rats decreased anxiety and regularly promoted mental and physical activity.

May aid brain health

Many neurological conditions, such as multiple sclerosis, Alzheimer's, Parkinson's, and encephalomyelitis, inflammation of the brain and spinal cord triggered by a virus infection, have been seen to find support and cure from the use of yarrow. Recent animal research noted that the severity of encephalomyelitis and brain inflammation and spinal cord and brain injury caused by it were decreased by yarrow extract. Plus, a rat study showed that the antioxidants of yarrow had anti-seizure benefits, rendering this herb a potential therapy for epilepsy patients. Additional rat experiments suggest that Alzheimer's and Parkinson's disease signs, such as memory loss and physical movement deterioration and muscle tone, can be avoided by this plant.

May fight inflammation

Although inflammation is a normal response of the body, chronic inflammation can damage cells, tissues, and organs. Yarrow may minimize inflammation of the skin and liver, which can help cure skin diseases, indications of skin aging, and non-alcoholic liver disease. A test-tube analysis showed that yarrow extract reduced inflammation and increased moisture in the skin. Other test-tube experiments show that this extract can decrease inflammation of the liver and control fevers.

How to add it to your diet

Yarrow comes in a variety of forms, like tinctures, powders, ointments, extracts, and flowers and dried leaves. By steeping 1–2 teaspoons (5–10 grams) in boiling water for 5–10 minutes, the leaves and flowers can be made into tea. The dried herb and also premade tea bags can be purchased from different health stores or online. Yarrow powder can also be added to smoothies, water, and juice. Bear in mind that there is inadequate data to set dose standards for yarrow tea and other products. Before consuming this herb, you should still refer to product labeling and contact a healthcare practitioner.

From online or indifferent health shops, you can purchase dried yarrow or premade tea bags. It also comes in other types, such as tinctures, ointments, oils, and powders.

Since ancient times, yarrow has been used medicinally, such as herbal tea. Research shows that wound healing, digestive problems, brain ailments, and other conditions can benefit from the plant compounds.

3.11 Basil

In the mint family, basil is a herb. It brings flavor to meals, and its nutrients can indeed offer health benefits. Basil is a delightful addition to soups, salads, and many Mediterranean dishes and is fragrant and simple to grow. The herb also provides oils and flavonoids that help protect the body from infection and disease. Basil has vitamin A, C and K, copper, manganese, calcium, iron, magnesium and omega-3 fatty acids that are beneficial. Basil can serve as an antiseptic for wounds and scrapes, as a healing herb, and it can give relief from headaches, flatulence, and loss of appetite. In a humid, sunny spot, grow your basil plant from seed, and keep the soil moist. An annual plant, basil is indeed very cold-sensitive. Cover it on days when the temperature drops to around 50 degrees. Snip the leaves for use. In many Mediterranean cuisines and particularly Italian ones, sweet basil (Ocimum basilicum) plays an important part. It forms a pesto base and adds to salads, spaghetti, pizza, and other dishes a distinctive taste. This herb is also featured in Indonesian, Thai and Vietnamese cuisine. Vitamins and a host of antioxidants can be provided by sweet basil in the diet. It has oil that may have therapeutic advantages as well. In several grocery stores, sweet basil is available, although other varieties have distinct tastes and fragrances. Tulsi, or sacred basil, is another form of basil (Ocimum sanctum). In Tamil and Ayurvedic medicines, which are mainly practiced in Southeast Asia, this plant plays a therapeutic role.

Health benefits

Basil consumption can help reduce oxidative stress. In the diet, as herbal medicine and as an essential oil, Basil can provide health benefits. Standard applications include, for example, the treatment of snakebites, colds, and irritation inside nasal passages, a frequent consequence of colds. Some macronutrients, such as calcium and vitamin K, are provided by Basil and several antioxidants. For instance, sweet Basil has a high concentration of eugenol, the chemical agent. This gives it a fragrance similar to clove. There are high concentrations of limonene in lime and lemon basil, which give them a citrusy scent. There are antioxidant properties of both eugenol and limonene.

Reduces oxidative stress

To remove free radicals from the body, antioxidants are necessary. Unstable molecules that form as a result of metabolism and other natural processes are free radicals.

As a result of smoking and certain dietary choices, they may also grow. Compounds that help remove these molecules from the body are antioxidants. Oxidative stress can occur if they build up instead, resulting in cell damage and, potentially, disease. Scientists have linked oxidative stress to rheumatoid arthritis, cancer, heart disease, diabetes, and other health problems. The body produces some antioxidants, but it also needs to absorb some from the diet. Anthocyanins and beta carotene are among the many antioxidants that are found in basil

Supports liver health

A 2015 research in rats found that antioxidants had a positive effect on liver health in a powdered formulation that contained tulsi, or holy basil.

Fights cancer

A study released in 2013 examined whether cancer could be inhibited by tulsi or holy basil. The researchers concluded that some forms of skin, liver, oral, or lung cancers could be prevented by the phytochemicals found in holy basil. This is achieved by increased antioxidant function, modifying gene expression, galvanizing cell death and delaying cell division.

Guards against skin aging

Sweet basil has properties that could help protect the skin from certain effects of aging, according to studies published in 2011. In the analysis, a basil extract was applied by the researchers to laboratory skin models. The findings indicated that it could increase skin hydration and minimize roughness and wrinkling using basil extracts in topical skin creams. While basil extracts can affect some doses, the skin would not generally benefit from eating basil. However, if a person eats them as part of a varied diet, the antioxidants in basil and other plant-based foods may well have a protective impact.

Reduces high blood sugar

To better control blood sugar levels, some traditional medicine practitioners commonly prescribe basil. Research in rats in 2019 showed that an extract of sweet basil leaves helps lower elevated blood sugar levels. The findings have shown that basil leaves can help to treat high blood sugar in the long term. If further investigations verify these results, basil extracts may prove beneficial for people with diabetes.

Facilitates cardiovascular health

A 2011 study reported observations that a sweet basil extract lowered elevated blood pressure briefly, likely due to the extract's eugenol content. Eugenol can block the body's calcium channels, lowering elevated blood pressure. In another study, 24 healthy participants were given either a placebo or a 300 milligrams (mg) capsule of dried tulsi leaf extract once a day. Those who took the tulsi extract had lower cholesterol and triglyceride levels after four weeks compared to those who did not. The researchers concluded that the extract might help reduce some cardiovascular disease risk factors.

Boosts mental health

The formation of free radicals in the body is caused by mental stress. The plant contains properties that can benefit:

- Easing stress, depression, and anxiety
- Increasing the capacity to think and to reason
- Preventing memory loss due to age
- Enhancing stress-related sleep and sex disorders

Some research reported findings similar to those of diazepam and antidepressant medications. Confirming these observations, though, would take further research. Consuming tulsi, for example, in a drink, is also doubtful to have the same effect as receiving an extract dosage.

Reducing inflammation and swelling

Oxidative stress could exacerbate inflammation, a condition in various diseases, like Type 2 Diabetes, cancer and rheumatoid arthritis. Researchers analyzed the anti-inflammatory effects of two sweet basil essential oil formulations in 2017. Basil oil can help cure different diseases that include inflammation originating from oxidative stress, according to their findings.

Fights infection

Various traditional medicine practitioners have been using basil as an antimicrobial agent, and some scientific evidence confirms this use. Scientists added sweet basil oil to separate strains of Escherichia coli in 2013. The bacteria came from patients with infections of the respiratory, digestive, genital, or skin, and hospital appliances. The findings revealed that the oil against these bacteria was effective. The study determined that some basil oil formulations may help cure or avoid certain causes of infection.

Nutrition

According to the United States Department of Agriculture, the table below shows some of the nutrients in 1 tablespoon of fresh basil weighing around 2.6 g. It also shows how much of each nutrient an adult needs, according to **the** ***2015–2020 Dietary Guidelines for***

Americans. Keep in mind; however, that needs vary according to sex and age.

Tips for use

Basil is a fragrant herb with a distinctive flavor that many people enjoy. The various types have different flavors. In cooking, sweet basil is the most popular variety in the U.S., but people also use lemon basil, clove basil, cinnamon basil, and other types. A person could:

- Sprinkle fresh, chopped basil over a pizza or into a wrap.
- Arrange some basil leaves over slices of tomato and mozzarella, then drizzle the dish with olive oil.
- Add basil to soups, tomato sauces, and stir-fries.
- Make a marinade with basil, olive oil, and chopped garlic.
- Add whole, chopped, or torn fresh leaves to a salad.

Or, try these recipes:

- Chili chicken with fried basil
- Fresh basil pesto sauce

- Pasta with tomato and basil sauce

Native Plants for Native Medicine

As they have been for centuries, the same good healers are many of the plant remedies commonly available in pharmacies and natural food shops. Although many of us are acquainted with botanical immune boosters such as echinacea and elderberry, or witch hazel's skin-soothing ability (to mention only a few), numerous other plants have strong medicinal roots and are native to North America. Since ancient times, people have needed plants to improve their lives and make the act of living a little more comfortable, not just for their survival. Here are the powerful plants whose conventional uses continue to educate and influence how we care for our diseases and encourage human health.

4.1 California Poppy

It is possible to medicinally use all parts of the California poppy plant, from its bright orange roots to its leaves, flowers and seedpods. The flowers were prepared by the Costanoan tribe members as a strong tea to clean their hair and kill head lice. The seeds were ground by the Ohlone individuals and combined with bear fat as a hair tonic dressing. Tribes in Mendocino's region juiced the roots to cure several different illnesses, from headaches to stomachaches to toothaches. Moreover, nursing mothers would wash their breasts with root juice to help dry the milk flow when it was time to wean their babies. Pomo women made a poultice and/or a strong tea from the mashed seedpods and applied it for the same purpose to their breasts.

4.2 Gooseberry & Currants

Currants and gooseberries have long been used medicinally by indigenous people of North America. To soothe inflamed throats, the Comanche people used berry tea as a gargle. A decoction from the root was developed by the Prairie Potawatomi tribe, which was good eyewash to extract foreign particles or soothe sore or irritated eyes. The Muscogee (Creek) tribe drank a powerful tea produced from the root bark to remove intestinal worms. To soothe painful and inflamed skin tissue, gooseberry juice was often applied to the skin as a wash.

4.3 Milkweed

The latex juice from the milkweed stems, plant tops, and the stem has been used for medicinal purposes by many native tribes. The Miwok people used latex to cure warts. A decoction of the dried plant tops was made by the

Cheyenne and used as an eyewash to treat snow blindness. Pleurisy root, also dubbed as butterfly milkweed (Asclepias tuberosa), was made into a cough remedy and was ultimately used by the people of Cherokee, Delaware, and Mohegan.

4.4 Nettles

The Hesquiaht and the Miwok people used the plant, often by whipping stems of fresh nettles over the infected body regions, to relieve muscle and joint pain. Transient burning and blistering were caused by the formic acid touching the skin, but it also generated a circulation rush to those parts. For problems such as arthritis, this increased circulation in the muscles and joints provided some permanent pain relief. Cherokee people and drunk prepared a tea from nettles as a stomach tonic. During gestation, the Cree Indians considered nettles an essential female herb.

4.5 Persimmon

Before the first frost, the Cherokee people gathered the fruits and turned them into an astringent herbal syrup to cure diarrhea.

The Choctaw sun-dried the fruit and, for the same reason, baked it into bread. The Catawba tribe developed a fruit poultice to cure warts and a decoction from the bark of the tree to use as a mouthwash for thrush (a type of fungal infection). To ease heartburn, the Rappahannock Indians used to chew the bark.

4.6 Spruce

In long, freezing winters, Native Americans knew that tea made from spruce needles helped people remain well. In Quebec City, Settlers started to suffer from scurvy in the 1500s (caused by a vitamin C deficiency). The Iroquois Indians shared with them this effective solution. In addition to curing them of scurvy, drinking spruce tea and spruce beer, dubbed Newfoundland spruce beer, became an essential preventive measure.

4.7 Willow

Along with many other tribes, the Choctaw and the Delaware Indians used peach leaf willow (S. amygdaloides) and other plants to make a toothbrush from a small willow twig.

Their teeth can be brushed, and the astringency of the tannins helped preserve good gums.

4.8 Yew

As a means of contraceptive, women of the Okanagan tribe and other northwestern coastal tribes consumed yew berries. To cure tuberculosis, arthritis and kidney failure, the Quinault people cooked the bark as a decoction and consumed it in very small quantities. The Cowlitz Indians developed a needle poultice and applied it to wounds topically. However, the leaves are not to be consumed orally since they are toxic.

Uses of Yew

In medicine and folklore, the yew has always occupied a special place. Being evergreen and renowned for its longevity, both death and immortality have been linked with it.

It has been recognized in the last decade that the pseudo alkaloids of different species of yew are effective antimitotic agents that are beneficial in some cancers that are highly resistant to other drugs. It is a slow-growing evergreen tree that can grow to 25 meters in height (80feet).

Its bark is rust-red, and the needle-like leaves are dark green. Paclitaxel is a drug extracted from the bark of the Pacific yew tree (Taxus brevifolia), the most well-known natural drug for the cure of cancer in the United States, and is used in the treatment of breast, prostate, and ovarian cancer, as well as Kaposi's sarcoma.

4.9 Chamomile

Another simple medicinal plant to grow at home is Chamomile that is quite popular as a soothing tea. Chamomile gives comfort to an irritated stomach, in addition to its soothing effects, which can relieve skin irritations. For decades, Chamomile has also been used as a soothing way to relax colicky infants. Chamomile plants like full sun and can grow to about 18 inches in height. It is easy to grow German Chamomile from seed.

Moreover, after the first season, the plants tend to self-sow freely. Within six weeks of planting, the beautiful daisy-like flowers emerge, supporting two plantings in one outdoor growing season. Cool, full sun and neutral climate favor German Chamomile in addition to mildly acidic, well-drained soil. Place the blooms to dry in a warm, dark place.

A common name for a large number of plants that look like daisies is Chamomile. To help people sleep and relax, these herbs have been used in the finest herbal teas. Chamomile contains coumarin, a drug that, much like aspirin, thins out the blood. This plant is indigenous to Europe and Asia but has now spread across the world. Native Americans have since been introduced to the plant, and they have immensely benefited from the plant. The plant holds substances that are so potent that pregnant women or women who are breast-feeding are advised against its use. Chamomile, since it has an anti-inflammatory effect, has also been as cosmetics. Did you know the Chamomile is also used for blonde hair enhancement?

Benefits of Chamomile

Chamomile is commonly used around the world and has many advantages and uses, as a muscle relaxant. This can assist with abdominal cramps, stomach pains, or muscle tension. Buy the herb and brew your tea. Many athletes have taken to chamomile following a tough workout to help calm the body. For most of the pains, two or three cups a day are adequate. The herb can also be used for the skin, and burns, asthma, and many other skin conditions can be healed. Chamomile has been used as a treatment for clearing acne and other skin irritations, as well as an anxiety remedy. The plant has oils that are very helpful to the human body, and its fragrance is popular. It has also been recognized that it is used to disinfect houses. To cope with digestive issues, as well as incense, the Native American herbal medicines used chamomile as a drink.

- Has many simple and stable applications
- Helps with headaches
- Nice to use with skin disorders

- Assists with cramps of all forms
- Has cosmetic features

Chamomile Uses

Chamomile may be used to produce tea, cream, or tablets for all sorts of other purposes. Tea can help with all types of things, primarily dealing with issues with the stomach. To cope with anxiety and heart attacks, numerous teas have been brewed with Chamomile. Chamomile has also been made into a cream that assists with issues with the scalp. You should apply the cream to help with bruises, wounds, as well as scrapes. The cream is also used for skin clearance, mostly for those with acne or eczema. Due to the oils, it contains, Chamomile has also been credited with minimizing unnecessary gas and bloating. It will help avoid a migraine before it even starts. Chamomile is a perfect treatment for migraines. Women who have had PMS or menstrual cramp issues will find chamomile tea a perfect and safe way to handle the said issues.

Pinyon

Pinyon is better known for its edible seeds. Although there are two pinyon species native to Utah, Colorado pinyon (Pinus edulis) and single-leaf pinyon (Pinus monophylla), Native Americans similarly use them. Pinyon has a broad range of medicinal applications. The pitch was used for various diseases, including wounds, some form of skin problem, digestive or intestinal disorders, infectious diseases such as colds, flu, tuberculosis, venereal disease, sore muscles, rheumatism, fevers, and internal parasites. It was also heated and subsequently applied to the face to remove excess hair or avoid sunburn. As an emergency ration, the inner bark was consumed or converted into an expectorant tea. To relieve fevers, the needles were chewed and swallowed to improve perspiration. To make a fumigant for earaches, buds were chewed and turned into a poultice for wounds or dried and pulverized. Making dyes or colors, gluing arrows, cementing turquoise jewelry, or waterproofing weaved water jugs or baskets were practical uses of the pitch. A tremendously important food source was pine nuts, and there were even more ways of consuming them than either raw or fried. They were mixed with berries and stored for winter use, made into cakes or gruel, mixed with yucca fruit pulp and made into a pudding, kneaded into seed butter, spread on bread, or made into hard dough, frozen, and eaten like ice cream. They may be ground into flour and rolled into balls. For added flavor, some tribes ground them with shells. Generally speaking, a strong pine nut harvest is only expected once every seven years. An outbreak of smallpox followed this, probably because several distinct groups gathered together to share the harvest and likely transmitted the disease. Practically every other aspect of the pinyon had used as well. Pollen has been used, often in place of cattail pollen, for ritual purposes. Since it was resistant to rot and wood-eating beetles, pinyon wood was valuable for house construction, and it was also used to produce useful things such as cradles, looms, saddle pieces, tools, and toys.

Juniper

Most of the medicinal uses of Juniper, unlike pinyon, were derived from infusions or boiling extracts of leaves, twigs, needles, or cones rather than from pitch. Nevertheless, with a list of disorders as long and variable, these preparations were used: renal complications, pneumonia, venereal disease, diabetes, cardiac problems, hemorrhages, stomachaches, vomiting, menstrual cramps, colds, fevers, smallpox, flu, cholera, tuberculosis, chickenpox, worms, swelling, rheumatism, burns, sore throats, hives or sores, and boils or slivers. To kill ticks on animals, a heavy decoction of the cones was also used. Bluish, berry-like cones with one or two seeds were boiled and eaten or dried and added to water for a drink or ground into a meal. They have been pierced and strung for beads as well. British Columbia's Okanagan-Colville tribe found the cones to be toxic and used them on bullets or arrowheads to kill people in warfare more easily, but they also made a drink from the cones and drank it in the sweathouse. Juniper bark served well as a torch. It was also well suited for storing fruit and covering floors, and thatching roofs for lining and covering pits. Juniper wood had many applications, as with other species, such as building lodges, corrals, fence posts, horse yokes, drums, flutes, spoked wheels used in a throwing game, bows, and bowls. The needles and boughs of Juniper had extra defensive powers over sickness, death, and sorcery. During epidemics, boughs were hanged around the house to keep away germs and were considered effective remedies to drive away bad spirits associated with death. For protection from grizzlies, hunters have even rubbed themselves with juniper boughs. For their holy, purifying smoke that could ward off disease, defend against ghosts, and eradicate the fear of thunder, the needles were burned ceremonially.

Douglas-fir

There were medicinal uses of all parts of Douglas-fir. Cuts, boils, other skin disorders, coughs or sore throats, including injured or dislocated bones, were cured by the pitch. It should be combined with oil and taken for abdominal discomfort, diarrhea, and rheumatism, among other illnesses, as an emetic (to induce vomiting) and purgative (a good laxative). It was also administered as a gonorrhea diuretic. The bark had antiseptic properties and helped with bleeding intestines and stomach, prolonged menstruation, and allergies induced by touching hemlock water. A strong general tonic and a remedy for paralysis are used through its needles. Bud tips for mouth sores are chewed. For colds, venereal disease, urinary disorders, or an emetic for high fevers and anemia, a decoction or infusion of young shoots was also used. Douglas-fir did not have as much fruit as some other trees, but the pitch could be chewed like gum or consumed as a sugar-like food, as in many other evergreens. The needles and young shoots could provide tea, and seeds were possibly used as a fruit, but they were not nearly as large and nutritious as the pinyon seeds. The wood found its way in such valuable tools as spear shafts, snowshoe frames, bows, tepee posts, and dugout canoes. Strong camping beds and sweathouse flooring were provided by Boughs. In basket making, twigs could serve as a coarse twine wrap, and pitch could be used for canoes as glue and patching material. To smoke buckskin, rotting wood was used, thereby retaining and dying it. For parts of the Douglas-fir, many tribes had separate ceremonial uses.

Ponderosa Pine

For sores and boils, aching backs and joints, sore eyes, earaches, and a general tonic, Ponderosa pine pitch was used medicinally. To speed up placenta delivery, hot needles were used, and a decoction was useful for coughs and fever. Boughs were used for muscle discomfort in sweathouses. To assist with hemorrhaging and high fevers, plant tops were used. Many tribes used the sweet inner bark for food. It could be eaten raw, rolled into balls for a tasty treat, baked into cakes, mixed with corn and meat and used to spice broth, or peeled off into strips and dried for later use as a highly nutritious food supply. It was obtained while the sap was running on cold, cloudy days, and various sources have compared the flavor to either sheep fat or lemon syrup. The seeds, either raw or fried, or dried and powdered and made into small cakes or bread, have also been used for food. Practical applications tended to outnumber the dietary and medicinal uses of ponderosa pine. The pitch can be used as a hair tonic, as a glue for the production of arrows and other items, and as a waterproofing agent for water jugs and moccasins. When out foraging, the bark was ideal for portable shelters or containers for sand painting pigments. The plentiful long needles could also be used to make baskets, insulate underground storage pits or pit house roofs, or provide a platform for roasting berries. A blue dye was produced using the roots, and the root fibers were used in basketry. The wood was useful for big roof timbers, fence posts, corrals, lodge sticks, dugout canoes, ladders, cradleboards, saddle components, and snowshoes.

Conclusion

The world cultures have concentrated and depended on conventional herbal medicine for centuries to fulfill their healthcare needs. The global market for herbal medicines is on the rise, amid the modern age's medical and technical advances. Currently, this sector is expected to gross over $60 billion annually. Some natural remedies can be more affordable and convenient than traditional medications, and since they comply with personal wellbeing principles, many individuals choose to use them. In their day-to-day life, Native Americans used a great number of herbs, and while most of these habits are no longer common, many ethnobotanical studies have introduced them to the world. While anthropologists have mainly concentrated on native applications of herbaceous and shrubby plants, various reports also show native uses of trees. Trees were used by Native Americans primarily for medicine, food, instruments, protection, and ritual aids. The needles of evergreens, for example, were widely used for tea.

Similarly, the pitch was chewed as gum, the inner bark was eaten for food and/or medicine, the wood was used for home and instrument building, and various parts were used for purification or cleansing. Similarly, the uses of these trees by various tribes vary considerably. Since ancient times, cultural health activities have been in place and continue to be essential means by which well-being is preserved and pursued. Traditional medicine is described by the WHO as the "total sum of knowledge, skills and practices based on theories, beliefs and experiences indigenous to different cultures, whether or not explainable, used in health maintenance along with in the avoidance, diagnosis, enhancement or treatment of physical and mental illness." The roots of Native American and Hispanic cultures are prominent in the Southwest, with traditional healing methods being common in both communities. Native American healing practices include herbal medicines to cure physical conditions; cleansing ceremonies in preparation for healing; and shamanism, based on the idea that spirits cause illness. Cultural healing techniques may be used by both Mexican Americans and Native Americans while still using Western medicine.

Nevertheless, you may wonder if herbal choices are safe. In a survival case, if you intend to use the herbs, learn to recognize them now so that you can identify them when you need them. If the Native Americans used them, maybe you too could use them safely and protect your life as a result.

NATIVE AMERICAN HERBAL REMEDIES

Traditional Herbal Remedies & Recipes to Heal Common Ailments

Introduction

Everyone is curious about how medicinal plants are used by native North American populations. The famous belief is that the central figure was the medicine man in the early Native North American indigenous community. However, this word may involve a broad range of activities, including a priest, a sorcerer, a quack, and even a doctor. The shaman was the priest's predecessor; the physician's predecessor was a lay healer, sometimes a woman. In some Native North American tribes, this division between the priest and healer was marked. Thus, the Ojibways had four shaman classes. The priests were highest in rank; then the "dawn men" who practiced a kind of medical magic; the seers and prophets were third; and ultimately the herbalists, who, in the context of being healers, were the real medicine men. Any or all of these were merged into one entity in other tribes, a forerunner of today's holistic treatment aimed at concurrently curing body, mind and soul. The knowledge and practice of medicine by the Native North Americans were not significantly different from their European counterparts when the European colonies were founded in North America in the 17th century. In both cases, the care of injuries caused externally was rational and always productive. Fractures, dislocations, burns, snake and insect bites, and so forth were included in this group. However, neither culture was able to treat most forms of prolonged internal illness where the trigger was not clear. As European nations expanded throughout North America, as part of their subduing the tribes, they attempted to eliminate Native American culture. The shaman was the primary obstacle to this, both as a priest and as a tribal chief. He or she was seen by Christian missionaries and leaders alike as antagonistic to foreign ideas and societies and was opposed. Yet, despite this, among the early colonists, native North American medicine greatly influenced therapeutics.

Colonial health professionals were not always physicians, especially in frontier regions. Today, there are also concerns about insufficient care by physicians and hospitals in many rural parts of the United States. The colonists resorted to the native North American herbalists, the "medicine men" or "medicine women," where there were no colonial medical practitioners or where their prescribed remedies had failed. Some of their treatments were unsuccessful, as in Europe, but there are many others that worked.

They had been discovered through

by casual observation, sympathetic association and by trial and error. But there was barely any method of standardizing decoctions and identical preparations, of course, and sometimes the specific batch had to be titrated against any patient's response. Nevertheless, an important collection of remedies was founded by the Native North Americans. About 170 preparations that were official in different editions of the United States Pharmacopeia or the National Formulary were used by the tribes in the present United States and Canada. Moreover, in the modern British Herbal Pharmacopoeia, the use of 25 percent of plants (more than fifty species) originated in North America, although they are now cultivated and used in Europe. Indian pinkroot (Spigelia marilandica), a Cherokee vermifuge, which was officially recognized in 1752 and included in the pharmacopeias of London, Dublin and Edinburgh, was one of the most important sources of early medicine.

At the beginning of the 17th century, nevertheless, sassafras bark was as commercially valuable as tobacco. Sassafras extract has been used in the treatment of rheumatism and gout as a febrifuge, carminative, and sassafras oil as a topical analgesic. At one time, wild cherry bark (Prunus virginiana and P serotina) was second only to home-medicated sassafras. The bark was applied directly to poultices and, as an injection, was used as an astringent in the treatment of coughs, colds, fever and cramps. As a sedative, narcotic, diaphoretic and emetic, Tobacco (Nicotiana tabacum) was legal in earlier editions of the USP. It has been used on crops as dust or an infusion, as an insecticide. Today, in reality, it is cultivated mainly for smoking. Cotton is indigenous to most of the subtropical countries. In the mid 16th century, Spanish explorers discovered that the North American species (G hirsutum) was grown by the Zui tribes in what is now western New Mexico; it is still the most commercially valuable species. Like tobacco, it is primarily cultivated for non-medicinal purposes as well. The fiber is still used for dressings, and as an emmenagogue and oxytocic, a decoction of the roots was used. Indian (or American) cannabis (Apocynum cannabinum), which is native to North America, should not be mistaken for Indian hemp (Cannabis indica). The American hemp fiber was used to make bags,

ropes and quilts, etc. The root was utilized as a diuretic and a cathartic. The most commonly used (natural) cathartic on earth is said to be Cascara (Cascara sagrada). An anonymous Spanish priest discovered the Native North Americans using it and was so struck by its mildness and effectiveness that he coined the botanical name "holy bark" (in Spanish). As a demulcent and emollient, slippery elm (Ulmus fulva) is still being used. It was also used by native North Americans for the prevention of coughs, colds and dysentery. The bark was used as a poultice in the treatment of bullet wounds during 18th-century military interventions.

The book will explain in depth the different treatments and the different kinds of problems that can be managed using Native American Herbal Remedies.

Conventional Healers and Healing

For a broad range of medicinal purposes, Alaska Native, Native American and all of the Native Hawaiian healers have a long tradition of using native or indigenous plants. Medicinal plants, along with their applications, are as diverse as the tribes that use them. Beyond their medicinal advantages, prior to Western contact, indigenous plants the staple diet of native people. Indigenous plants are central to current generations' attempts to enhance dietary well-being. In Hawai'i, by restoring the function of indigenous foods, the 'Waianae Diet' and 'Pre-Captain Cook Diet' seek to minimize empty calories, fat, and additives and encourage a healthier, more balanced diet. Similar ventures emphasizing traditional foods have been conducted by Alaska Natives and numerous Indian tribes. Food is medicine.

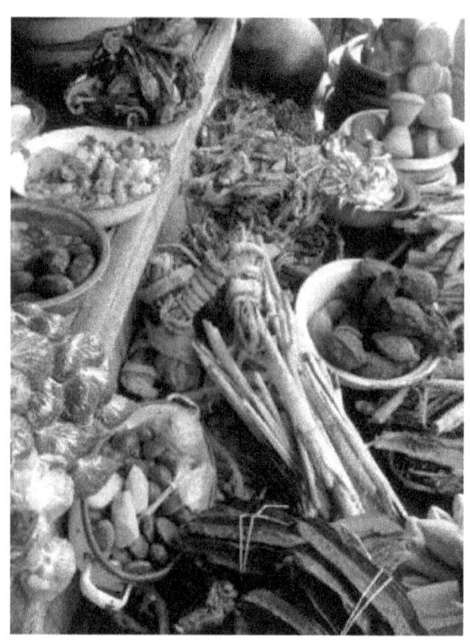

In the United States, there is an increasing interest in medicinal botanicals as part of complementary medicine. In particular, Native American societies are becoming conscious of using herbals by both practitioners and consumers; many botanicals marketed today as dietary supplements in the United States were used for similar purposes by Native Americans. However, these supplements constitute only a small number of >2500 different vascular taxa plant species and >2800 species of all taxa known to have been coveted by the indigenous inhabitants of the North American continent for their medicinal properties.

Plants and Native Americans

In the medicinal practices of many, if not all, Native American populations, plants play a significant role. Plants are therefore used not only in the diagnostic process but also in the procedures for physical and ceremonial purification that typically precede ceremonies and in the act of healing itself. Of the >17000 plant species that make up the North American flora, more than 2500 members of the vascular taxa and >2800 of all taxa were used by various Native American societies for medicinal purposes to some degree continue to be used. For at least a century, the compilation of knowledge regarding the use of specific plants as medicine has been in progress. The resulting knowledge was collected in book form in 1986 and, more recently, in a database on the Internet. Yet, new medicinal plants and plant use already included in these databases continue to be discovered by ethnobotanists. Native Americans have documented unique uses of medicinal plants, and, surprisingly, several different tribes in diverse areas of North America have often used the same plant components. Examination of plants that are used as medicines by original North American inhabitants revealed that, as shown by the widespread use of certain plant families and the virtual exclusion of others, the choice of the medicinal botanicals was not random but highly limited. Several lines of evidence indicate that, in the context that Western science uses that word, Native Americans took botanicals as medicine. For example, for the treatment of various illnesses, Native Americans used different plant parts, mixed multiple botanicals for particular therapeutic reasons, and they are recognized toxic plants as both actual poisons and for medicinal purposes. However, we should stress that plants' use for the treatment of specific symptoms often requires a spiritual aspect because it is the strength, the "spirit," of the plant that is thought to have the therapeutic effect.

1.1 Rules used for collecting the plants

For a plant to have "power," it is important to follow certain rules while collecting the plant. The instructions recorded from such culturally and geographically distinct tribes like the Iroquois of the Northeast and the Salishan of the Northwest are surprisingly agreed upon. The significance of gathering plants in the morning is emphasized in both tribes; tree bark is to be extracted from the eastern side of the tree, a tobacco offering is to be made, and prayers need to be said. Such specifics are not always mentioned regarding the collection process or, perhaps, more importantly, the particular plant component used and the method of its preparation. This lack of knowledge and the fact that the medicinal use of plants by indigenous residents of North America has usually, transcended the mere physical contribution to the lack of literature dealing with the medicinal properties.

Many of these botanicals can easily be found in health food stores and, to a growing degree, supermarkets and pharmacies. Some of the species used by Native Americans are also native to other parts of the world (e.g., Sambucus nigra, Sambucus racemosa, and J. communis); others have been introduced by indigenous North American populations to European settlers and have subsequently become common in Europe [e.g., species of Echinacea and Lobelia inflata]. In exchange, settlers from other continents intentionally or unintentionally carried some native botanicals, resulting in the subsequent use by Native Americans of some foreign plants (e.g., Tanacetum vulgare and Urtica dioica).

Therefore, what little research exists on species used by the original inhabitants of North America primarily comes from other countries where the same species have been used, mostly for the same therapeutic purposes as Native Americans had already recorded. However, variations in the concentrations and ratios of chemical constituents, subsequently in biological activity, will also occur in plants grown in the same vicinity, depending on the environmental conditions; more variability will be introduced by the time of production, storage and processing the extraction method.

1.2 Some Selected plants and their uses by Native Americans

Genus and species and part used	**Indication**	**Societies that used the plant**
Echinacea angustifolia		Cheyenne, Dakota, Fox, Kiowa, Montana Indians, Omaha, Pawnee, Ponca, Teton Sioux, and Winnebago
Infusion of leaves and roots	Taken for sore mouth, gums, or throat	
Plant	Antidote for many poisons and venoms	
Root	Antidote for snake bites; used in medicine for stomach	

	cramps and bowel pain	
Ground roots	Chewed for coughs and sore throat	
Smashed roots	Applied as poultice to snake bites, stings, and septic diseases	
Juice	Used to wash burns and to relieve pain	
Plant	Used in smoke treatment for distemper of horses	
E. pallida		Cheyenne and Dakota

Decoction of roots	Taken for rheumatism and arthritis, smallpox, mumps, and measles; taken as vermifuge; used as a wash for burns and fever	
Roots	Chewed for colds	
Poultice of roots	Applied to inflammation	
Plant	Antidote for snake bites	
E. purpurea Moench		Choctaw and Delaware-Okl

Root	Chewed for cough and dyspepsia	
Tincture of root	For cough and dyspepsia	
Infusion of root	Taken for gonorrhea	
Urtica dioica L.		Chehalis, Cherokee, Cowlitz, Iroquois, Klallam, Kwakiutl, Lummi, Ojibwa, Potawatomi, Quileute, Quinault, Samish, Shuswap, Shagit, Shokomish, Snohomish, Squaxin, Swinomish, Tainarna, and Wet'suwet'en
Whole stalk	Used to whip person with	

	rheumatism or paralysis	
Infusion of stalks	Rubbed on body for soreness and stiffness	
Infusion of nettles or crushed leaves or tips of plants	Taken before or during childbirth	
Infusion of roots	Taken for treatment of intermittent fever	
Infusion of pounded roots	Taken for rheumatism	

Decoction of stems and roots	Used as sweat bath for rheumatism	
Boiled rhizomes	Used as a general medicine	

Native American Herbal Remedies for Scores of Ailments

Native Americans have used herbs for thousands of years to not only cure the body but also to purify the spirit and bring harmony to their lives and their surroundings. A study of oral practices suggests that they learned by observing sick animals about the healing abilities of herbs and other plants. Prior to the first contact between Europeans and the tribes, there were no written reports of medicinal usage by America's indigenous people. However, this changed as Native Americans shared with the new settlers their understanding of how to use nature's drugs. Although there were scores of herbs and plants that were used as remedies by Native Americans, one of the most sacred was tobacco, which was used for curing various illnesses, as well as in rituals and ceremonies.

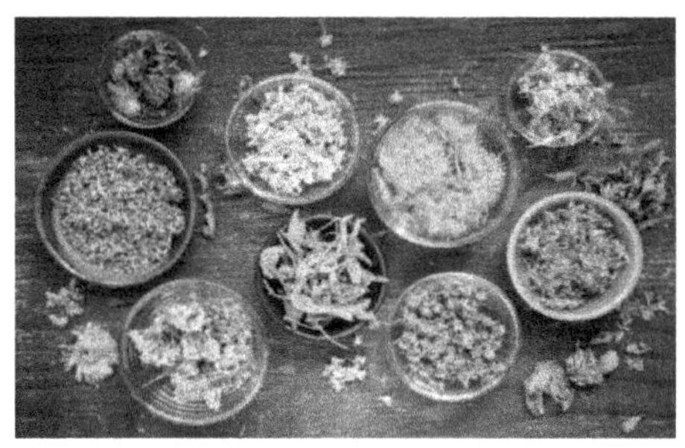

It was solely smoked and not mixed as it is today with any additives. Sage, which was said not only to cure many problems of the lungs, stomach, colon, kidneys, liver, skin and more, was another very significant herb for the Native Americans; it was often thought to protect against evil spirits and to draw them out of the body or the soul. While there are numerous and diverse lists of medicinal herbs that could be carried in a Healer's medicine bundle, those most commonly used were often carried, such as common cold remedies. A selection of herbs used mostly by Native Americans that are helpful for different ailments is given below. It also includes herbs used for many of the illnesses of today.

2.1 Cardinal Flower

Formally, this plant is called Lobelia Cardinalis. This plant is native to the Americas, starting from southeastern Canada south through all the eastern & southwestern United States, Mexico & Central America. It usually has bright red flowers. The root was used by Native

Americans to cure bowel problems, typhoid, worms, epilepsy, cramps, and syphilis. For colds, bronchial symptoms, croup, nosebleeds, fever, headache, and rheumatism, leaf tea was used. A poultice of the roots was used on sores to heal and applied to the head to alleviate headache pain. The dried leaves were smoked by the Penobscot tribe as a replacement for tobacco. It is regarded as potentially toxic as a member of the Lobelia family, but the degree of toxicity is uncertain. It has been acknowledged that the plant's sap causes skin irritation.

2.2 Catnip/Catmint

It is officially called Nepeta Cataria and is also known by Catswort. Although it is native to Europe, Asia, and Africa, it is now popular in North America. Because of its calming properties, the plant has a long history of medicinal use and has also been known to have a slightly numbing effect. Used in poultices, it is eaten in teas and smoked. Fresh or dried stems and leaves are used to make aromatic herbal tea, which has been found to be beneficial in treating digestive system disorders, reducing fever, treating colds, influenza, and infant colic. In the treatment of restlessness and nervousness, it has also been found to be useful. Salves are manufactured externally from the leaves. Then they are applied to injures, mainly black eyes. Raw young leaves having mint-like taste, have also been used in salads and cooked foods as a seasoning. It was found to inhibit insects, mice, and rats when the oil was isolated from the plant.

2.3 Cat's Claw

Officially referred to as Uncaria Tomentosa, it is also known as Cat's Nail. It has been used for medicinal purposes as a general health tonic, anti-inflammatory agent, contraceptive, gastrointestinal and urinary tract issues, breathing issues, diarrhea, rheumatic disorders, acne, and diabetes for more than two thousand years as a tropical vine that grows in the rainforests and jungles of South America and Asia. Current studies also indicate that it can have beneficial effects on prostate disorders, PMS, Aids, diabetes, chronic fatigue syndrome and cancer care and improve the body's immune system.

2.4 Cayenne

It is also commonly known as Red Pepper, Chili Pepper, Hot Pepper, Pimiento, Mexican Chili, Tabasco Pepper, and many other local names. It is officially referred to as Capsicum. It is native to the Americas, where it has been grown by people in the tropical regions for thousands of years and is now cultivated worldwide. It has been best known for treating circulatory and digestive problems and was used as both a supplement and for medicinal purposes. Chronic nerve pain, rheumatism, arthritis, shingles, diabetes, heart disease, gastrointestinal ailments, varicose veins, headache, menstrual cramps, and asthma were additional disorders for which it was used. For throat pain, it was often used as a gargle. It was applied externally to wounds to improve blood flow and to numb the pain. More recently, it has been used to lower cholesterol and blood pressure.

2.5 Chamomile

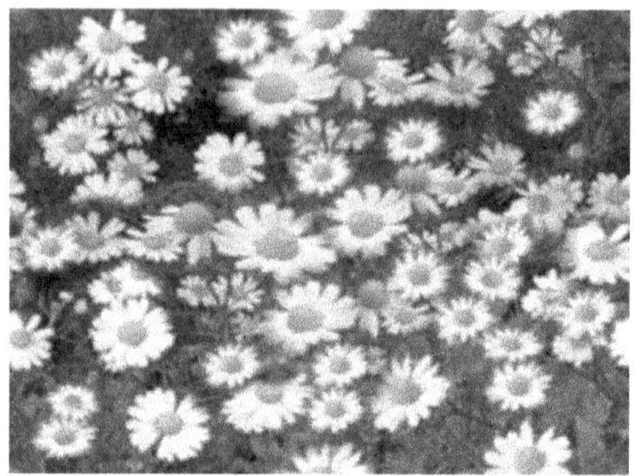

They are mostly recognized for their capability to be made into a tea that is widely used to assist with sleep. They are a common name for many daisy-like plants. They are also believed to treat stomach and intestinal cramps, problems, nausea, stomach, and flu, including gynecologic complaints, PMS, and cramps. It is also an excellent agent for calming and well balanced for babies and kids.

2.6 Chasteberry

Chasteberry is the fruit of Chaste tree, known as Vitex Agnus-catus. It has been used for more than thousands of years to help alleviate the effects of menstrual problems and improve breast milk production. It was probably used by monks in the Middle Ages to suppress sexual appetite and maintain purity, hence the name, and was also known as chaste tree berry, vitex, and monk's pepper. It is now clear, however, that the herb does not affect the drive for sex. In teas for PMS, berries and flowers were used to alleviate menopausal symptoms, for breast pain, acne, and fertility. Today, for bone strength and as an anti-inflammatory and epilepsy, it has also been effective. Chasteberry should not be used by pregnant or breast-feeding women.

2.7 Chokecherry

It is also named Western Chokecherry, Black Chokecherry, and Wild Cherry and is formally known as Prunus Virginiana. You can find varieties all over the United States and Canada. The tree has long been used as a source of food and medicine by various tribes, including the Miami, Mohawk, Huron, Penobscot, Delaware, Cree, Ojibwe, Iroquois, Chippewa. It was considered one of the most significant native drugs in early American medicine, ranked along with Sassafras. For later use, the berries were gathered and dried, and the tree bark was used in the treatment of smallpox, scurvy, chest and throat pain, lung hemorrhage, cough, colds, intestinal inflammation, diarrhea, stomach cramps, cholera, digestive disorders, gangrenous wounds, sores, pain, serious burns, and wounds. They learned about the health properties of chokeberry from the Indians when Europeans arrived in America and started to use it to treat cough, cold, consumption and malaria, burns and wounds. There are small variations between the varieties, ranging from red to purple to black, including the color of the fruit. While the berries are edible, caution should be used because if eaten in large enough amounts, the pit can be poisonous.

2.8 Chlorella

It is a genus of single-celled green algae that has shown promise of anti-tumor properties and efficacy in cancer prevention, support for the immune system, weight management, high blood pressure reduction, cholesterol-lowering and wound healing acceleration.

2.9 Chickweed

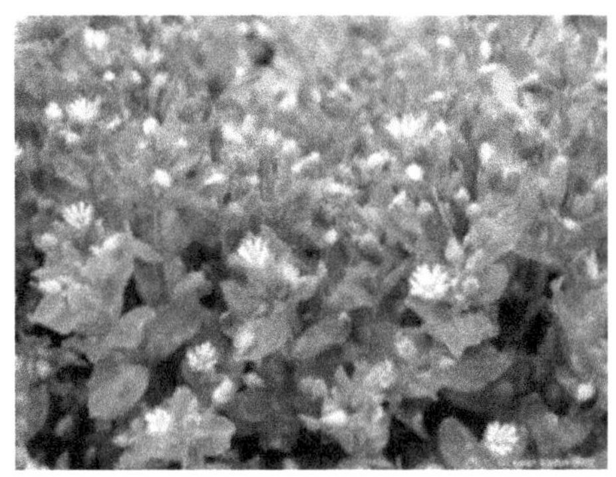

The likely origin is Eurasia, but it is nowadays made all around the world. It is formally known as Stellaria Pubera and Stellaria Media. It is common in North America, from the Brooks Range in Alaska to all south points. They have also been used for food and medicine, also known as Star Chickweed, Common Chickweeds and Mouse-ear Chickweed. The whole plant, rich in vitamins and minerals, has been used as an antihistamine, astringent, diuretic and expectorant, and treat symptoms of constipation, urinary tract, cough, and cystitis and kidney. Poultices have been used externally for treating roseola, wounds, rheumatic pains, ulcers, eczema, skin problems, cuts, mild burns, and rashes.

2.10 Coltsfoot

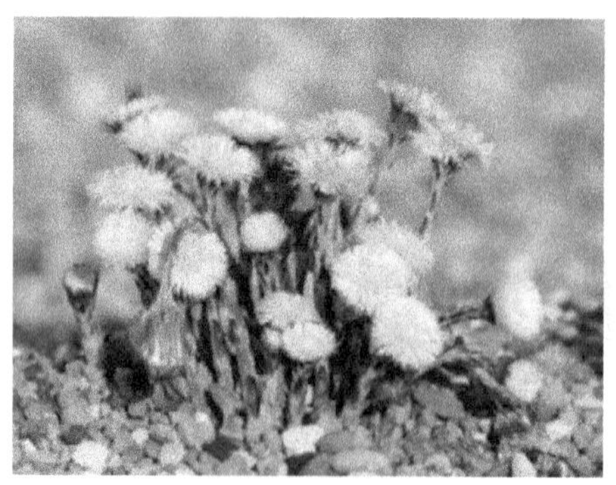

This dandelion-looking herb, scientifically known as Tussilago Farfara, has been used medicinally across the globe for hundreds of years. Pedanius Dioscorides, a pharmacologist and Greek physician, who lived from 40-90 AD, prescribed it for cough and asthma. It was native to several areas in Europe and Asia and was known by many other names, including British Tobacco, Coughwort, Bullsfoot, Butterbur, Flower Velure, Horsehoof, and others. It was brought by early colonists to the Americas and now grows in North America, northward from Kentucky and Tennessee to Ontario and Quebec in Canada, and in Minnesota and Washington, west of the Mississippi River. Usually, the leaves were smoked for whooping cough, cough, bronchitis, and other respiratory problems. Crushed leaves were often used for diarrhea, flu, pleurisy, inflammation, sore throat, fever and indigestion in teas and tonics. Various skin diseases, inflammation, insect bites, burns, skin ulcers and sores, crushed leaves and flowers were also used actively.

2.11 Cotton

Cotton, from the genus Gossypium, is native to subtropical and tropical regions around the world. This includes Africa, the Americas, and India. In the treatment of urinary problems, roots, leaves, and seeds have been used to support the contraction of the uterus after childbirth, prolonged menstrual bleeding, wound and burn healing, dysentery, and diarrhea. To alleviate the pains of labor, the Alabama and Koasati tribes produced a tea from the plant's roots.

2.12 Creosote Bush

The plant is formally named Larrea Tridentata, and many refer to it as a medicinal herb called "chaparral." In the deserts of the south and the western US, it is common. Native Americans of the Southwest made tea from the leaves and used it to remedy respiratory disorders, chickenpox, sexually transmitted infections, tuberculosis, dysmenorrhea, and snakebite. Regretfully, the US Drug Administration has issued alerts about the health hazards of ingesting chaparral.

2.13 Damiana

The small aromatic shrub is known officially as Turnera Diffusa and is native to Central America, southwestern Texas, southern California, Mexico, South America, and the Caribbean. A stimulating effect on libido has long been acknowledged as the major benefit of its use, and its use as an aphrodisiac has persisted into modern times. It has also been used in the treatment of impotence, asthma, depression, menstrual problems, nervousness, anxiety, and constipation to raise energy and improve digestion.

2.14 Dandelion

It is known to most individuals as a common plant, officially called Taraxacum Officinale, but to herbalists because of its many culinary and medicinal uses. Its leaves are rich in vitamins A, B complex, C, and D. Its leaves are also rich in minerals such as iron, potassium, and zinc and have also been used to flavor food and teas, its roots in coffee, and its flowers to make certain wines. Dandelion roots and leaves have been used in herbal medicine to treat liver disorders, kidney failure, swelling, skin problems, heartburn, and disturbed stomachs. The Pillager Ojibwas drank a tea of the roots for heartburn, and a tea of the leaves was drunk by the Mohegan tribe as a general health tonic. It was used by the Chinese to treat stomach problems, appendicitis, and breast issues (like inflammation or lack of milk flow). In Europe, herbalists have integrated it into remedies for fever, boils, eye diseases, diabetes, and diarrhea. Today, dandelion roots are primarily used for liver and gallbladder functions, as an appetite stimulant, and for diuretic and digestive aid.

2.15 Dogwood

This flowering tree native to the U.S. is scientifically known as Cornus Florida and can be traced from Maine to Florida and west to Minnesota, Kansas, and Texas. Its berries, inner bark and twigs have long been used in Native American remedies with many other common names, including Cornelian Tree, American Dogwood, Boxwood, Budwood, Flowering Dogwood, Green Ozier and others. It was mainly used internally to treat malaria, cough, pneumonia, colds, and diarrhea and boost appetite and digestion. Poultices have been used externally for treating ulcers and sores. In the early 19th century, it was recorded that the white teeth of Native Americans in Virginia were extraordinary. Twigs were used as chewing sticks, that was like toothpick and a brush for chewing. The Iroquois were famous for using the twigs in a gonorrhea tonic, and the Cherokee chewed the headache bark and used a bark decoction to treat childhood problems such as worms, measles, and diarrhea. They also developed poultices for wounds and other skin conditions, which were also used. The bark was used in enemas by the Menominee, and the Arikara combined the bearberry to produce sacred tobacco. During the Civil

War, this was used for malarial fever commonly and chronic diarrhea in the South.

2.16 Geranium

There are around 200 varieties of geraniums among the Pelargonium species found all over the world. Stork's Bill and Scented Geranium are among the other common names. Scented geranium leaves were used in traditional folk medicine in teas to treat ulcers, headaches, etc. The Cherokee were recognized in Native American medicine to have boiled geranium root along with wild grape that was utilized to rinse the mouths of those children who were affected by thrush. For diarrhea, the Ottawa and Chippewa tribes boiled the whole geranium plant and then drank the tea.

2.17 Ginkgo Biloba

In Korea, China, southern France, and in the eastern and southern United States, Ginkgo Biloba trees are believed to be one of the most ancient trees still in existence. The trees can live as long as 1,000 years, and food and medicinal treatments have long been made and used from their leaves. Thanks to its beneficial effects, it is most widely used for treating the elderly as a circulatory aid for disorientation, memory loss, depression, headache, Alzheimer's Disease, dementia, tinnitus, and vertigo.

Effective for circulation problems, ADHD, cramps, and as an antioxidant. It has also been found to be effective in high blood pressure.

2.18 Goldenseal

This herb from Buttercup family, scientifically known as Hydrastis Canadensis, and is also known as Orange Root, Yellow Root, Ground Raspberry, Puccoon, and Wild Curcuma. It was historically used by native people to treat skin disorders, stomach problems, liver conditions, diarrhea, as a stimulant, and eye irritations. It was also used by people native to southeastern Canada and the northeastern United States. It is also known that the large rootstock was pounded by the Cherokee with bear fat and smeared it as an insect repellent on their bodies. The herb was introduced by the Iroquois to early settlers for medicinal use. It has also been successfully used for the treatment of infections of the mucus membranes, along with the mouth, urinary tract, sinuses, intestines, throat, stomach, and vagina, as well as mild wound healing, flu, colds, bladder infections, and inflammation of the sinuses and chest. Pregnant women should not take Goldenseal.

2.19 Hawthorn

Of the Crataegus species, as far back as the 1st century, Hawthorn has been used to treat heart disease. It was used by American doctors at the beginning of the 1800s to handle circulatory disorders and respiratory diseases. Traditionally, berries have been used to combat heart issues ranging from irregular heartbeat, chest pain, arterial hardening, and heart failure to high blood pressure. The leaves and flowers are used medicinally today, and there is clear evidence that Hawthorn is capable of treating mild to severe heart failure. Hawthorn contains antioxidants as identified in animal and laboratory studies.

2.20 Hellebores

Commonly referred to as Hellebore, there are approximately 20 species of these flowering plants native to Eurasia, many of which are poisonous. It has long been used in old herbal remedies, also known as Bugbane, Devil's Bit, Earth Gall, Indian Pinch, Itchweed, and Tickleweed, but is no more used today as the herb has been found to be severely toxic and has many serious side effects, including in therapeutic dosages. American Hellebore has traditionally been used internally for the treatment of influenza, peritonitis, epilepsy, pain, asthma, cold, cholera, croup, consumption, dyspepsia, flu, headache, hypertension, herpes, gout, inflammation, whooping cough, sciatica, shingles, toothache, tumors, rheumatism and typhus. It was used as a gargle for infections of the throat and tonsillitis and skin irritations externally. It was claimed that the Cherokee used the green Hellebore to relieve the pains of the body.

2.21 Hops

The female flower clusters, typically known as strobiles or seed cones, have long been known as the flavouring and stabilisation agent in beer. They have been native throughout Europe and Asia. However, they have also been used for a number of conditions in traditional herbal medicine. It has long been used as a digestive aid, and to also relieve pain, and as a sleep aid because of its bitter ingredients. Often used alone, but often used to relieve anxiety, restlessness, to soothe muscles, most frequently used with other herbs. Within a pillow, a sachet packed with hops was often used in popular folk medicine, where the herb's aromatic properties can help a person fall asleep. The Mohegan tribe is known to have prepared a sedative remedy that was applied to toothache in Native American remedies; the Dakota people used tea to alleviate digestive organs pain, and the Menominee tribe treated a similar hop species as a general panacea.

2.22 Horehound

This plant is from the Mint family, technically called Marrubium Vulgare, is native to Europe but is now naturalized in North and South America. It has long been used to treat stomach disorders, as well as a variety of other illnesses, with many common names, including Eye of the Star, Bull's blood, Poison Tobacco, Houndsbane, Hog Bean, Devil's Eye, and others. As a cough suppressant and expectorant, Horehound has medicinally substantiated its importance and is still used in producing cough drops. Other applications include constipation treatment, tuberculosis, gastric disorders, painful menstruation indigestion, flatulence, bronchitis, colds, nausea, whooping cough, and a stimulant for sedation and appetite. Externally, it has been used to treat skin conditions, sores, abrasions, and cleaning agents for wounds. It should be used carefully by people with gastritis or peptic ulcer disease.

2.23 Horsemint

This is a species of the Mint family, officially known as Mentha Longifolia, native to Europe and Asia, and has long been appreciated for its antiseptic properties and effect on digestion. In teas and tonics, leaves and flowering stems have also been used to cure inflammation, fever, headache, chills, colic, flatulence, congestion, menstrual disorders, cough, colds, and urinary infections tract. As a stimulant and to induce labor, it has also been used. It has been used externally for swelling, sores and superficial wounds. To alleviate nasal and bronchial congestion, leaves and stems were often added to boiling water, and the vapors were inhaled. The Catawba tribe pounded, and steeped fresh horsemint leaves in cold water in Native American Medicine and drank the infusion to ease back pain. Horsemint was used by other tribes for fever, inflammation, and chills. It should not be used by women who are pregnant.

2.24 Rabbit Tobacco

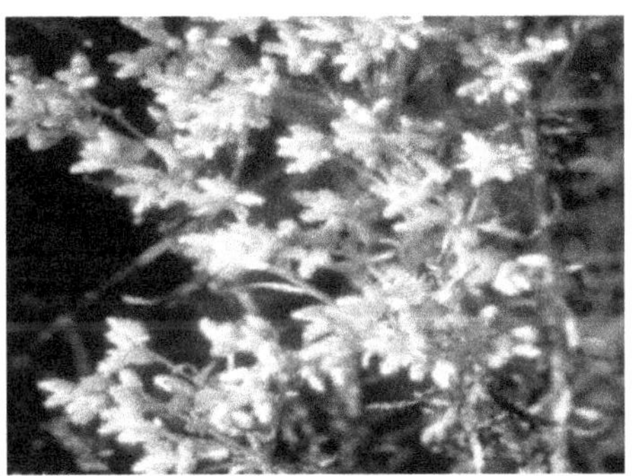

Also recognized as Sweet Everlasting, Cherokee Tobacco, Indian Posey, Old Field Balsam, Cudweed, Poverty Weed, Fussy Gussy, and Sweet White Balsam, it is formally called Gnaphalium obtusifolium. In pastures, woodland, prairies, and thickets in the eastern states, east of Colorado, it grows almost everywhere. It has long been used by Native Americans for a number of medicinal purposes using the stem, leaves, and flowers for treating asthma, diarrhea, cough, colds, flu, bronchitis, pneumonia, as an insect repellant, sleep aid, and many other purposes. It was mostly smoked by both Native Americans and early settlers in place of tobacco and did not contain nicotine. The smoke was thought to have held for many Indians a mystical or magical influence. The Cheyenne also dropped leaves on hot coals, and it was known to have been used by the Cherokee in sweat baths. The Creek used it as a cold remedy, as a poultice for mumps in which it was applied to the throat, and as a sedative.

Furthermore, the Koasati for fever, a psychological aid and the Menominee for headache when dried leaves were steamed in the form of anodyne for "foolishness." Also some tribes believed the smoke had a vital power that could awaken the unconscious or paralyzed. It was used on bruises and skin and mouth sores when a poultice was made. The Cherokee also developed a herb salve that blended with lard and rubbed on the chest to alleviate congestion and encourage sweating. The plant's juice had both a reputation as an aphrodisiac and an anti-venereal potion. It induces sleep, helps migraines, sinus problems, cough, asthma, stomach problems, is a mild sedative of the nerve, and increases appetite.

2.25 Ragleaf Bahia

This flowering plant belongs to the daisy family and is also widely known as yellow ragleaf or yellow ragweed. It is known officially as Bahia Dissecta and was also referred to by the Navajo tribe as Twisted Medicine. It was used by many tribes as a contraceptive in teas. It is indigenous to the southwestern United States as far north as Wyoming and also northern Mexico.

2.26 Framboise

The leaves and fruits, which are identified by Rubus Idaeus and Rosaceae's names, respectively, have a long history of use in pregnancy to reinforce and tonify the uterine tissue, support contractions, and check any bleeding during labor. It is useful as an astringent in a wide variety of situations, particularly diarrhea, and to relieve mouth problems, like mouth sores, gum bleeding, and inflammation. It is also used as a gargle to assist with sore throats. For digestive problems and moderate nausea, new or dried leaves were often steeped in tea.

2.27 Saltbush

There are many species of this herb, and it is also known as Orache. It is officially known as Atriplex. It comprises several desert and seashore plants that are highly tolerant of the soil's salt content. Their name is derived from the fact that in their leaves, they retain salt. For a number of health problems, different forms have long been used, including discomfort, rashes, sores, stomach ache, spider and insect bites and more. It was often used for water purification. The Hopi were known to burn and inhale the smoke for treatment of epilepsy and often used it for ritual medicine in kiva fires; the Paiute to boil the leave that they used for sore muscles and aches a poultice was applied for colds to the chest. The Navajo were believed to have been using leaves for pain, cough, stomach issues, and as a toothache treatment, in addition to using them for insect bites.

2.28 Sarsaparilla

The perennial trailing vine with those prickly stems is scientifically called Smilax Aspera and Smilax Regelii. It is native to Central America and is most widely known for its use in soft drinks. It has been used for several centuries around the world and was introduced into European medicine in the 1400s by interaction with the indigenous tribes of South America. It has many useful applications in herbal treatments to help digestion, pain, blood washing, asthma, wounds, colds, impotence, gonorrhea, hypertension, rheumatism, fever, cough, skin disorders, leprosy, and cancer, even including treatment for syphilis. It has anti-oxidant effects, much like many other plants. In conjunction with Sweetflag, the Penobscot was thought to use the pulverized dried sarsaparilla roots as a cough remedy.

2.29 Sassafras

These small trees or shrubs native to Eastern North America, from Maine to Ontario, south to Florida and Texas, are officially known as Sassafras Albidum. Sassafras was used widely by Native Americans for food and medicine long well before European settlers arrived, and its bark became one of the New World's first exports. In early American folklore, the tree's sweet fragrance was associated with healing and protection from evil forces by explorers and settlers, and extracts of the bark and roots quickly became a panacea elixir actively sought by Europeans. It has been used for the treatment of fever, measles, chickenpox, flu, as a blood purifier, colds and as a cure over the years.

2.30 Savory

Officially known as Satureja, Savory is a genus of rosemary and thyme-related aromatic plants from the Mint family. There are approximately thirty species called savories, including the Summer Savory, Mountain Savory and Winter Savory. It has long been considered that summer savory, which is more highly valued as a spice and as well as a folk medicine, functions as an aphrodisiac. It also has a wide range of applications, including assisting the system and curing flatulence, diarrhea, cough, and colic in herbal remedies. It was effectively used on the chest for curing congestion.

2.31 Saw Palmetto

This small palm, known as Serenoa Serrulata in scientific terms, grows in the south-eastern parts of North America. Its berries have been enjoyed by both humans and wildlife for a long time. For a wide variety of purposes, including food, Native Americans have been utilizing saw palmettos; the leaves were used to weave baskets and ceremonial dance fans. The heartwood of the palms was used as well as pounded into flour for traditional medicinal purposes. It has been used in diarrhea, stomach pain, digestive support, prostate health, cough, breathing, inflammation, sexual vigor, congestion and appetite enhancement.

2.32 Skullcap

This perennial herb in the mint family, officially called Scutellaria Lateriflora, is native to North America and grows in Canada and the northern United States. Also recognized as Hoodwort, Blue Skullcap, Virginian Skullcap and Crazy Dog, it has promoted the reproductive system. It was historically cultivated and used for menstrual cycles by Native American women. The herb has been used by several tribes in purification ceremonies. The Iroquois used a root infusion to keep the throat clean, while some plants were used by other tribes as bitter tonics for the kidneys. Its effectiveness against stress relief, help for the nervous system, insomnia, tension, and restlessness have also been found. It is an effective medicinal plant, anti-inflammatory, abortifacient, used as a sedative to treat epilepsy, hysteria, anxiety, infections of the throat, headache, discomfort, anxiety, seizures, and more. The Skullcap should not be taken by pregnant women.

2.33 Slippery Elm

The Slippery Elm formally called Ulmus Rubra, is a genus of elm native to eastern North America, from east to southern Quebec, south to northern Florida, and west to eastern Texas, from southeast North Dakota. The tree had many typical Native American uses, including inner bark fiber for yarn, bowstrings, cords, clothes, and more. For various purposes, the wood was used, and for medicinal purposes, the bark along with leaves in washes and teas. Digestive diseases, gastrointestinal problems, arthritis, sore throats, ulcers, gout, stomach ache, intestinal worms, cough, bronchitis and other respiratory irritations were also included in the medications. Whole bark was often used as an abortifacient but often had severe repercussions. It was also used for the treatment of skin disorders, vaginitis, hemorrhoids, toothaches, and spider bites.

2.34 Spearmint

Officially known as Mentha Spicata, known as (Spear Mint or Spearmint) is a mint plant native to much of Europe and Southwest Asia. For the treatment of bronchitis, chills, cramps, fever, chronic gastritis, headache, indigestion, common cold, morning sickness, motion sickness, nasal inflammation, nausea, and painful menstruation, a medicinal herbal tea was made of fresh or dried leaves that had a very good and refreshing taste. It has been used externally for bruises, swelling, muscle soreness and rheumatism.

2.35 Stevia

Common to subtropical and tropical regions from western North America to South America, it is a genus of around 240 species of herbs and shrubs in the sunflower family. The species Stevia Rebaudiana has long been used as a sweetener and in the treatment of heartburn, obesity, flatulence, diabetes, and hypertension, commonly known as Sweetleaf and Sugarleaf.

2.36 Stiff Goldenrod

It is formally known as the Rigidum Oligoneuron, and also known as the Rigid Goldenrod Prairie Goldenrod. It has been found that the leaves and blossoms are an effective antiseptic, astringent and prevent bleeding. In the prevention of all kinds of hemorrhages, it has long been a valuable solution. The flowers were also ground into lotion and used for the treatment of bee stings by Native Americans.

2.37 St. John's Wort

St. John's Wort is most widely used as an antidepressant, legally known as Hypericum Perforatum, and also known as Tipton's Plant, Chase-devil, or Klamath weed. It has also been used to treat joints problems, decrease swelling, sprains, cramps, fractures, varicose veins, signs of menopause, and anxiety.

2.38 Stoneseed

Also commonly known as Gromwell, this plant genus belonging to the family Boraginaceae is technically known as Lithospermum Officinale. For a long time, the mature seeds have been ground into a powder and used as a sedative to treat bladder stones, arthritis. Some Native Americans have used the roots as a contraceptive, such as the Shoshoni. In treating eruptive diseases such as smallpox, measles and itching, syrup from the root and stem decoctions were also used.

Medicinal Plants that Native Americans Used daily

For their medicinal plant knowledge, Native Americans are renowned. After seeing animals consume certain plants when they became ill, it is rumored that they first began using plants and herbs for healing. The medicine men used to select every third plant they encountered to protect these plants from over-harvesting. The Native Americans had a holistic vision of life, and a person had to have a sense of mission and follow a just, harmonious, and happy course in life to be safe. They felt that such diseases were life lessons that the person needed to understand and shouldn't intervene. The Native American interpretation of the many plants and herbs they have used for thousands of years has been used by many modern treatments and medicines.

3.1 American Indian practice of Medicine

For an American Indian, the sense of the word medicine is somewhat distinct from that usually held by western cultures. Medicine involves many theories and concepts for many of these American Indians, instead of remedies and care alone. From tribe to tribe and in various cultural areas, there are differences in the healing process. There are several processes, though, which are almost universal. Prayer, chanting, poetry, herbalism, counseling, and ritual are conventional forms of treatment.

3.2 Herbs use as medicine

It is assumed that men's herbs drew their strength from the ceremonies carried out to make them strong. The core of their herbal conviction was "Like cures like." Yellow plants are ideal for jaundice; red plants are beneficial for blood. The organ of the body that it is meant to heal may imitate any part of the plant. The use of worm root for the treatment of snakeroot for fits, worms, elm bark, owing to its slippery nature, is used for bloodroot and bleeding lungs is used to suppress bleeding. The Indians have often claimed that the system benefited from such roots or plants because they are repulsive and detrimental to the demons that cause illness in the host body. There are scores of plants that were used as medicines by Native Americans. When we emphasize medicinal plants common to our North American homes, Mother Earth Living's dual focuses on environmental wellness, and local food converge. Each part of the planet is blessed with its healing plants in harmony with nature's fascinating abilities to provide for our well-being. A lot of common plant awareness in North

America comes out of the American Indians, who have counted on medicinal plants for much healthcare.

Nonetheless, understanding American Indian herbal medicinal usage is complex. Firstly, medicinal plants' use differed extensively among the various tribes, and knowledge of the uses of the plants is also traditionally protected. Given below is a description of various herbs that were used by native people for the treatment of different diseases.

3.4 Sumaca

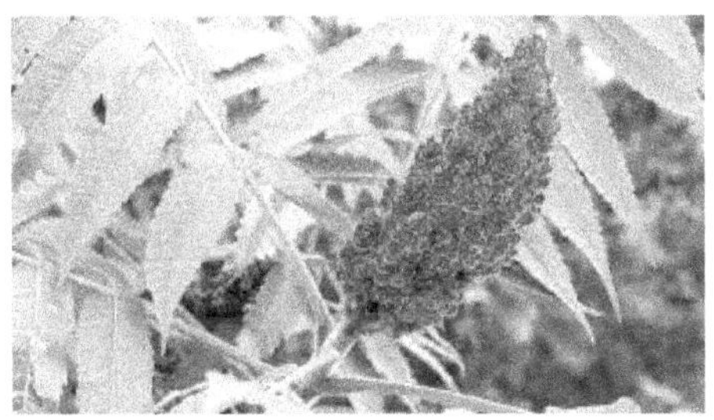

This plant can be used in various herbal treatments, but it is one of the few plants used by healers to cure eye problems. As a gargle to treat sore throats and is also taken as a treatment for diarrhea, a sumac decoction was used. The berries and leaves were mixed in tea or turned into a poultice to ease poison ivy to control fever.

3.5 Blueberry

The Cherokee used this herb to relieve a disturbed stomach. For treating diarrhea and calming sore tissues and joints, they used blackberry tea. Blackberry root combined with honey or maple syrup will produce an all-natural cough syrup to cure sore throats. They used to chew the leaves to soothe bleeding gums. Often, this plant is ideal for improving the whole immune system.

3.6 Rosemary

This plant was considered sacred by Native American tribes. They used it mainly to alleviate swollen muscles as an analgesic. This herb strengthens memory, relieves pain and spasms in the body, and helps the circulatory and nervous systems. The immune response is also strengthened, and indigestion is treated.

3.7 The Mint

To soothe digestive issues and help an irritated stomach, the Cherokee used to produce a mint tea. They also formulated a leaf salve to alleviate itchy skin and rashes.

3.8 Red Clover

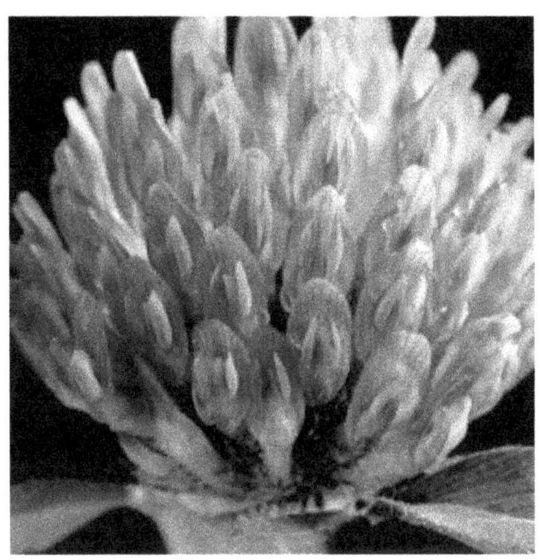

Healers have used this herb for the treatment of asthma and respiratory problems. The latest findings have found that by improving breathing and lowering cholesterol, red clover helps reduce heart disease.

3.9 Black Gum Bark

For making a mild tea from the twigs and black gum bark Cherokee is used, for alleviating chest pains.

3.10 Cattail

There are about 11 species, officially called Typha, mainly occurring in wetland ecosystems in the Northern Hemisphere. Several names, including Bullrush, Reedmace, Punks, and Corndog Turf, are also well known. These were also used to build a supply of food that was refined into flour that was nutritious and energy-rich.

From mature male flowers, pollen was also gathered and used as a flour substitute or thickener. Various species are used in Native American herbal medicine in poultices applied to burns, inflammation of wounds, sprains, boils, and swelling.

It has been used internally for stomach cramps, kidney stones, whooping cough, gonorrhea, cysts, and diarrhea. Specifically, in various treatments, the Apache used pollen; it was used by the Dakota, Ponca, and Pawnee for dressing burns and scalds; the Algonquin for treating infection; the Cahuilla for bleeding wounds.

In their Sun Dance ritual, the Cheyenne were even known to have used leaves. This is one of the most popular survival plants used for food and as a protective medicine by the indigenous people. Since it is a meal that is quickly digestible, it helps to recover from sickness. It can be found in different dishes.

3.11 Pull Out a Sticker (Greenbriar)

This root tea has been used to purify blood or to alleviate joint pain. A salve was made from bark and leaves mixed with hog lard. This was used to treat mild sores, burn and scalds.

3.12 Hummingbird Blossom (Buck Brush)

To cure mouth and throat problems and cysts, inflammation, and fibroid tumors the Native Americans used this herb. To assist in healing burns, sores, and cuts, it can be turned into a poultice. Using the roots of this herb, a diuretic may be produced that stimulates kidney function. This unique plant was used as a substitute for black tea by the early colonists. The latest findings have shown that hummingbird blossoms effectively treat elevated blood pressure and blockages of the lymph system.

3.13 Ferocious Rose

This herb was used by Native Americans as a preventive and a treatment for moderate common cold. The tea stimulates and is a gentle diuretic for the bladder and kidneys. For a sore throat, a petal infusion was used.

3.14 Saw Palmetto

The plant was used for food by Florida's tribal tribes, such as the Seminoles, but medicine men used it as a natural cure for abdominal pain. It also encourages digestion, lowers inflammation, and promotes appetite.

3.15 Sage

This small evergreen shrub is technically known as Salvia Officinalis and is sometimes referred to as garden sage and common sage. Many Native Americans consider Sage holy because of its powerful purifying forces. It cures and cleanses the body and mind of evil spirits by creating harmony. For thousands of years, people have been cooking with sage, and, like other culinary herbs, it has long been believed to be a digestive aid and stimulant of appetite as well as a cure for a variety of other medical disorders, like flatulence, intestinal cramps, bloating, spasms, coughing, diarrhea, colds and flu, scratches, bruising, premature menstruation, tuberculosis, stomach ache, extreme suddenness. It has also been good with menstrual cramps, halting the development of breast milk, signs of menopause, cough, throat infections, and dandruff. As a spice, sage is widely used.

3.16 Ginger

This herb is used by healers to cure earaches and ear infections. They also used the rootstock for making a gentle tea to improve the digestive system and alleviate bloating. It also assists in nausea and bronchial infections.

3.17 Slippery Elm

Using the inner bark, the Native Americans fashioned bowstrings, cord, yarn, and clothes. Tea was made using its bark and leaves to soothe toothaches, lung irritations, skin problems, stomach pain, sore throats, and even spider bites.

3.18 Lavender

This herb has been used to treat insomnia, nausea, depression, headache, and exhaustion by healers. Antiseptic and anti-inflammatory effects are found in the essential oil. To soothe bug bites as well as wounds, infusions may be used.

3.19 Prickly Pear Cactus

This is another herb used both as a meal and as medicine. Native Americans developed a poultice as an antiseptic and for healing cuts, burns, and boils from mature pads. Tea was made to cure diseases of the urinary tract and to aid the immune system. The study now suggests that the prickly pear cactus helps lower cholesterol and reduces cardiovascular disease and diet-related diabetes.

3.20 Honeysuckle

This herb has been used by Native Americans to cure asthma as a natural remedy, but it has various healing uses, including rheumatoid arthritis, mumps, and hepatitis. It also assists with infections of the upper respiratory tract, such as pneumonia.

3.21 Ashwagandha

Due to its many rare medicinal applications, this plant was an important plant for healers. It addresses bone fatigue, stiffness and muscle weakness, missing teeth, loss of memory, and rheumatism. And, it can be used as a sedative. If it increases vitality, it has an overall rejuvenating impact on the body. It is also essential to use the leaves and root bark as an antibiotic. It tends to minimize swelling if turned into a poultice and treats discomfort. When using this herb, caution is recommended as it is poisonous.

3.22 Mullein

It was a tobacco-like plant that was used mostly to treat respiratory disorders. To relieve swelling in the joints, feet, or arms, the Native Americans made concoctions from the roots. Officially known as the Verbascum genus and sometimes known as velvet plants, these flowering plant species are native to Europe and Asia and were first introduced by Europeans to America. A tobacco-like weed has a long tradition of use as a medication for the treatment of asthma and respiratory diseases and is one of the oldest herbs. The smoke from smoldering mullein leaves and roots was frequently inhaled by Native Americans, including the Menominee, Woodland Potawatomi, Mohegan, and Penobscot, to alleviate asthma attacks, chest pain, and other respiratory disorders. The roots can be turned into a warm decoction to soak swollen feet, minimizing swelling in joints or other places, which can soothe sore tissues. It is especially useful for the membranes of the mucosa. Sweetened syrup from the boiled root was used by the Catawba Indians, given to their children for cough. For a moderate sedative, a tea may be made from flowers. In the treatment of ear infections, extracts made from plant flowers are used, and one species, called the Great Mullein, is used as a herbal cure for sore throat, cough, and lung diseases.

3.23 Licorice Root

For flavoring candies, meats, and drinks, this root is famously used. Yet healers have also used it to cure digestive problems, bronchitis, food poisoning, and constant tiredness.

3.24 Uva Ursi

It is also known as Bearberry and Beargrape, owing to the bear's affection for the fruits of this herb. This herb was used by Native Americans mostly to cure diseases of the bladder and urinary tract.

3.25 Devil's Claw

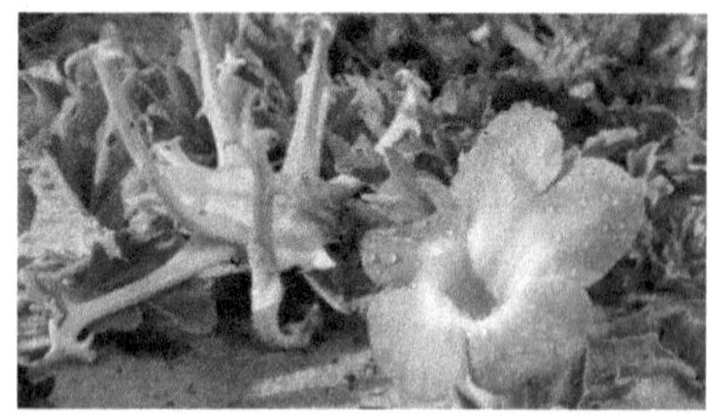

The Native Americans used it to remedy different illnesses, from curing fever to calming skin conditions, improving metabolism, and treating arthritis, while the name suggests it as a poisonous herb. While a concoction made from the plant roots prevents swelling and helps with joint disease, arthritis, gout, back pain, cough, and sores, tea may minimize the symptoms of diabetes.

3.26 Barberry

Anthropologists claim that it acts as a spiritual force or a preventative or cure of disease in a ceremonial activity or sacred object, especially by Native Americans. It is the most frequently prescribed treatment in the homeopathic medicine system for kidney pain and kidney stone removal.

3.27 Candle bush

Cassia alata Fungal infections such as ringworm are treated with leaves or sap. They include chrysophanic acid, a fungicide. It is also used to cure a wide variety of illnesses, including digestive disorders, fever, asthma, snake bite and venereal diseases, in addition to skin diseases (syphilis, gonorrhea).

3.28 Horsemint

A long history of use by many Native Americans, including the Blackfeet, Ojibwa, Menominee, Winnebago and others, as a medicinal herb. Used with skin diseases and minor damage infections caused by severe flatulence.

3.29 Cascara Buckthorn

This tree's charred, aged bark has been used continuously by native and European settlers as a natural laxative remedy for at least 1,000 years.

3.30 The Wormseed

Wormseed was used by the Maya of Central America for centuries to expel worms, and thus its name. The Aztecs used the herb to treat dysentery and asthma. The herb for poultices was used by the US's Catawaba people to detoxify snake bites and other poisonings.

3.31 White Hellebore

It is an extremely poisonous plant that has been extensively used by various indigenous North American Indian tribes who have used it mostly externally to treat wounds and discomfort.

3.32 Greek Valerian

Range: Northeastern United States, Georgia to the south and Minnesota and Oklahoma to the west. Native Americans used the root for piles or hemorrhoids to cure eczema, to trigger sweating and vomiting (inflammation of the epidermis).

3.33 Elder berries

It was used by Native North American tribes to treat a wide variety of symptoms such as cold, intake, headache, indigestion etc. In certain folk medicine cultures, all aspects of the elderberry plant are considered and recognized as a beneficial curing plant.

3.34 Angélica

It is originally from eastern North America. In Arkansas, Angelica was held in high regard by Indians, who often kept it in their medicine bags and combined it for smoking with tobacco. It relieves menstrual pain, decreases menopausal complications, manages colds and other coughing issues, avoids arthritis, and battles some cancers.

3.35 Pipsissewa

It is known that almost a dozen native tribes have used Pipsissewa as medicine. The application varies from the treatment of backache, sore eyes, gonorrhea, blisters, sore muscles, swelling of the leg and foot, etc. It is considered to be a blood purifier and to facilitate internal healing.

3.36 Balsam Fir

It was used by North American Indian tribes as an antiseptic curing agent and was externally applied to cuts, sores, bites etc. It was used to relieve headaches as an inhalant and was also taken clinically to treat colds, sore throats and multiple other symptoms.

3.37 Arrow Wood

In a decoction for cramps, the Ojibwa and Menominee Indians use the inner bark. In preparing a tea to drink to induce vomiting, Ojibwa also combines arrowwood and the bark of the alder (Alnus incana).

3.38 Bloodroot

The root's red juice was a very common cure for sore throats, respiratory disorders, and skin growth among the Plains Indians. For rheumatism, asthma, bronchitis, lung ailments, laryngitis and fevers, American Indians used the root.

3.39 Echinacea

Its popular names are Purple coneflower and Echinacea purpurea. Echinacea purpurea Moench is its botanical name. In American folk herbalism, Echinacea is one of the most commonly known herbal products. Echinacea was used widely for centuries by herbalists, and American Indians in North America achieved fame in Europe in the 1900s. One of its key uses, while many of its past uses have been linked to topical treatments, is to support better immune function. It is also one of the most commonly available nutritional supplements and continues to focus on clinical research in natural food stores. With heavy concentrations in Kansas, Arkansas, Oklahoma and Missouri, Nine plants are native to the United States and Canada. These species are perennial members of the sunflower family.

3.40 Black Cohosh

Its common name is BlackCohosh. Other names include rattle snakeroot, black bugbane, black snakeroot, bugwort, rattle root, rattleweed, squawroot, rheumatism weed. Actaea racemosa is its botanical name. Black cohosh, native to many parts of Canada and the United States, is a flowering perennial. It thrives in coastal forests and areas of substantial biodiversity. In the United States and Canada, the vast majority of the world's black cohosh is developed and grown. With a stem clustered with tiny white flowers, the plant grows between 3 and 6 meters tall. Between late July and September, the medicinal roots are best collected. For American Indians, who used it for a number of illnesses, it was a popular herbal remedy. The name derives from the Algonquian people, refers to the rhizome's feeling, which means rough. The name 'bugbane' was given because the flowers have such a strong odor, and they have been used to repel insects effectively. Black cohosh is commonly used to improve women's health and is licensed for premenstrual pain and distress associated with regular menstruation by the German Commission E. In supporting balanced menopause, black cohosh is sometimes utilized. It is used as a medication for disorders caused by lack of estrogen, such as menopause-related depression. This is backed up by the clinical experience of European practitioners. Clinical experiments suggest that black cohosh, either functioning as a moderate estrogen or regulating estrogen production in the body, has a calming effect on hormone production. For that reason, in herbal formulations for controlling female hormones, black cohosh is often used, especially those used to minimize hot flashes, which can occur when estrogen levels drop too low. Commercial herb formulations, available in the United States, are widely prescribed in Europe and are endorsed by several test-tube studies and a few human studies. In one randomized, double-blind trial, a standardized black cohosh extract was taken by 110 menopausal women who complained of adverse symptoms and who had not taken estrogen substitution therapy for at least six months. The women were less stressed and had fewer hot flashes than those in the placebo group, researchers reported.

3.41 Cranberry

Cranberry is its common name. American cranberry and large cranberry are the other names. Vaccinium macrocarpon is its botanical name. One of the most versatile antibacterial herbs is also a popular accompaniment to the American Thanksgiving meal. Cranberry is also anti-asthmatic and diuretic and provides side benefits in preventing urinary tract infections outside its conventional application. With nearly 98 percent of the world's production grown in the northern U.S. and Canada, Cranberry is a fruit native to North America. As for its medicinal and nutritious qualities, the indigenous Americans and colonists mutually valued cranberry. Cranberries are a high-value crop, ranked 40th in the USDA National Agricultural Statistical Service's recorded sales of all cash crops. The powdered berry is best for medicinal use. In sugar-free teas, it can be encapsulated or added. Many of the products on the market are freeze-dried and typically contain an anti-caking agent to avoid solidification.

Wards off urinary tract infections.

Several studies have confirmed that cranberries help avoid urethra and bladder infections. In one study of older people, cranberry juice, relative to placebo, decreased the number of bacteria in the bladder. Another research found that younger women who took cranberry capsules with a history of regular UTIs had reduced UTIs compared to those who took a placebo. Studies show, though, that cranberry does not function until you have a UTI.

Prevents ulcers.

Two studies have shown that cranberry may also inhibit stomach walls from attaching to the bacteria Helicobacter pylori. H. Pylori may cause stomach ulcers. Hence cranberries can play a part in stomach ulcer prevention.

Prevents cancer.

Some test-tube and animal studies indicate that cranberry may help stop cancer cell growth.

Fights viruses

Cranberry can help fight viruses in test tubes.

Fights bacterial illness.

Cranberry has demonstrated the efficacy of checking common forms of bacteria, like Escherichia coli (E. coli) and Listeria monocytogenes.

American Ginseng

American ginseng and Xi yang shen are the famous names. Panax quinquefolius is its botanical name. Ginseng is generally used for three separate herbs: American ginseng (P. quinquefolius), Asian or Korean ginseng (Panax ginseng) and Siberian ginseng (Eleutherococcus senticosus), the first of which has much of the same effects but belongs to a distinct genus of plants.

American ginseng is planted from Quebec to Florida in the whole eastern seaboard of North America. American ginseng has' cooling' properties and is known for its thirst-quenching effects, unlike Asian ginseng, which has' warming' properties. American Indians used it as a preventive measure in the same manner as the Chinese. It became a large business when it was first uncovered that ginseng grew wild in North America.

The American folk hero, Daniel Boone, was recognized as a fur trader, but he made a fortune trading wild-harvested ginseng. Most of the ginseng research has concentrated on the Asian variety, not the American variety. Both plants possess similar properties and are often used by herbalists interchangeably. Ginseng for invigoration and fortification has been approved by the German Commission E during times of need.

In healthy people, it has been shown to increase reaction time and focus. It has been shown in older adults that ginseng promotes healthy aging and memory. Ginseng is often referred to as an "adaptogen," meaning it is an herb that helps the body cope with different forms of stress, but there is little empirical evidence to explain the advantage of adaptogens. American ginseng is effective in improving the immune system and as an antioxidant in laboratory experiments in animals. Other experiments indicate that there could be medicinal capacity for inflammatory disorders in American ginseng. The following conditions have been the subject of research:

Diabetes

Several human trials indicate that in people with type 2 diabetes, American ginseng decreases blood sugar levels. The effect was shown both on blood sugar fasting and on glucose levels postprandial (after eating). One research showed that persons with type 2 diabetes who consumed American ginseng before with a high-sugar drink had a lower increase in blood glucose. Other findings indicate that North American ginseng reduces complications linked to diabetes, including improvements in retinal and cardiac function, by minimizing stress.

Cancer

It has been shown that American ginseng prevents tumor growth. Researchers discovered American ginseng had potent anti-cancer effects in one laboratory experiment on colorectal cancer cells.

Colds and flu

People consuming the American ginseng-containing medication Cold FX for four months had fewer colds than those taking a placebo in two trials. There were shorter symptoms for people who had colds than for those who had a placebo.

ADHD

A study suggests that American ginseng, along with Ginkgo biloba, may help treat ADHD.

Immune system

Some scientists claim that American ginseng strengthens the immune system, which may, in principle, help the body combat illness and infection. Several clinical trials have found that the efficiency of cells that play a role in immunity is improved by American ginseng.

Cognition

A study discovered that daily consumption of American ginseng improved cognitive function in mice.

3.42 Saw Palmetto

Its common names are Sabal palm and Saw palmetto. Serenoa repens is its botanical name. Saw palmetto, specifically concentrated in Florida and a few neighboring areas, is a small species of palm native to the Southeastern United States. The plants normally attain between three and six feet in height because they typically grow prostrate, reaching up to 15 feet on the occasional occasions that they grow upright. Saw palmetto plants could live for several years, and it is estimated that the oldest plants in Florida are between 500 and 700 years old. Saw palmetto grows during the summer and through October in sandy soil, yielding medicinal fruit. When fully mature, the fruit is bluish black. With a taste that is described as slightly soapy and acrid, it has a distinctive, sweet fragrance. Saw palmetto berries were used in Florida as a food source and a general tonic for American Indians and were consumed to stave off starvation by early American settlers. One of the first to note the beneficial impact the fruit had on grazing animals was American botanist John Lloyd, concluding that it could benefit humans. In the 1950s, the herb dropped out of favor when science did not account for the berries' observable behavior. Today, saw palmetto is among the herbs most widely used and researched to facilitate good functioning of the prostate.

Advantages

For more than 100 years, extracts of saw palmetto fruit had been used to treat prostate disorders, especially benign prostatic hyperplasia or BPH. BPH is characterized by a benign enlargement of the prostate (noncancerous) and is considered to affect more than half of men older than 50. It induces weak urinary flow that can trigger various symptoms, including urinary discomfort, painful urination, elevated urination frequency, and more. The use of standardized extracts of saw palmetto is confirmed by more than two dozen randomized clinical trials, the bulk of which were performed in Europe. Head-to-head clinical trials have reported that saw palmetto is as successful, with fewer side effects, as an ancient medicine in relieving BPH symptoms. The findings of the first U.S. clinical study were published in June 1999 on saw palmetto.

For six months, 44 men diagnosed with BPH got a saw palmetto extract or placebo. Prostate tissue size in patients treated with saw palmetto has been reported to have reduced from 17.8 percent to 10.7 percent, with almost no reported side effects. UCLA urologist Leonard Marks, the lead researcher, said, "Saw palmetto extracts appear to be a fair treatment choice for individuals with uncomplicated symptomatic BPH.

3.43 Beeswax

For centuries, beeswax has been used for all kinds of purposes, from embalming, candles, ointments, cosmetic items and more, taken from the honeycomb of bees. It also provided the foundation for many healing salves in fold medicine. In the early seventeenth century, honey bees were imported to North America, and Native Americans named them 'white man's flies' because their appearance suggested a nearby colonist colony.

However, for many hundreds of years, the Americas' indigenous peoples have used wild bees in their products. When combined with spices and as a balm for wounds, it was and is still used for producing medical ointments. Blood vessels have also been shown to dilate, thus improving blood flow. Beeswax can be used only outwardly.

3.44 Black Gum

officially known as Nyssa Sylvatica, from southern Ontario south and New England to central Florida and eastern Texas, the tree is native to eastern North America.

It is also frequently referred to as Black Tupelo, Pepperidge, or either Gum or Tupelo. Native Americans have used its fruit, bark, and roots as a bath, as well as in decoctions to trigger vomiting, remove worms in kids, and cure eye problems. To ease chest pressure, Cherokee healers used a gentle tea made from small bits of bark and twigs.

3.45 Black Raspberry

It is also identified as thimbleberry, wild black raspberry, black cap, blackcap raspberry, and scotch cap. It is formally known as Rubus Occidentalis. It has been found that the shrub's roots, which are boiled into tea or chewed, are cathartic and efficient in curing gonorrhea, cough, and toothache.

They were sometimes used for sore eyes, ulcers, boils, and sores as a wash. The root bark was boiled by the Pawnee, Omaha, and Dakota tribes to cure dysentery. In the care of bowel problems, extremely astringent leaves were used. In the treatment of whooping cough, a decoction of the roots, stems and leaves was used.

3.46 Blue Cohosh

This flowering plant is grown in hardwood forests from Manitoba, Canada, and Oklahoma east to the Atlantic

Ocean, traditionally called Caulophyllum Thalictroides, known as squaw root and papoose root.

The root in tonics and teas has long been used by Native Americans to treat dropsy, rheumatism, colic, hiccough, cramps, epilepsy, women's fertility disorders, uterine problems, and to stimulate labor and relieve childbirth pain. Many Native American tribes and later European herbologists and mid-wives used Blue Cohosh for abortive and contraception purposes combined with other herbs and remedies.

3.47 Blue Spruce

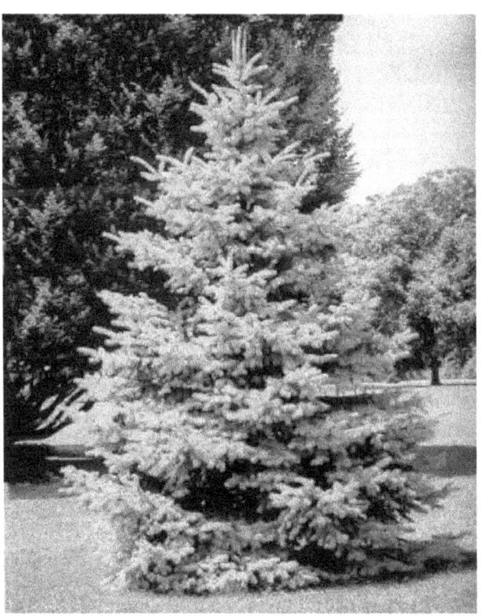

The Colorado Blue Spruce, one of the most common ornamental conifers, with its silvery blue-green coloring and perfect Christmas tree shape, is a truly majestic sight. In 1862, the Colorado blue spruce was first spotted on Pikes Peak, and its fame soon spread. It is one of the most regularly planted landscape trees today. It is not only stunning, but it has long been used for medicinal purposes by Native Americans. This tree is used as a traditional medicinal plant and a ritual object by the tribes of the Navajo and Keres, and twigs are offered as gifts to bring good fortune. It is said that the infusion of needles in a warm bath relieves the effects of rheumatism. For the prevention of colds or gastrointestinal ailments, various parts of the tree have been used. Spruce oil is obtained from spruce plants, bristly, needle-like leaves, and twigs, with which natives are used to curing skin issues such as boils, burns, skin irritation, sores, and wounds in ointments and salves with honey and alum. The spruce balsam was often chewed like chewing gum and spread as caulking or glue. In treating respiratory problems, bruises, burns, and swelling, its medical applications persist today; discomfort associated with arthritis, bone pain and pain in the joints, and more. Blue Spruce's various ingredients have also been used as a disinfectant, furniture cleaner, air freshener, and insecticide in homes.

3.48 Boneset

Officially known as Eupatorium Perfoliatum, it belongs to the asters' genus and comprises 60 species. It has also been called ague grass, feverwort, thoroughwort, or snakeroot, native to temperate regions of North America. While it is toxic, it was used to cure colds and fever by the Iroquois, Cherokee, Delaware, Mohegan, and Menominee. It was used as a laxative by Alabama with stomach aches and the Cherokee. It has also been useful in treating dengue fever, asthma, infectious disorders, migraines, intestinal worms, flu, measles, and diarrhea, and is rich in niacin, magnesium, and calcium and phosphorus. Generally found in tea, the possibly toxic contaminants would be removed by dried leaves rather than fresh leaves. Caution is recommended that liver injury can be caused by radioactive substances. Side effects cause muscle tremors, fatigue, and constipation.

3.49 Broom Snakeweed

It is native to the west and southwest parts of the United States, formally known as Gutierrezia Sarothrae, and is sometimes called snakeweed. It was used for various therapies by Southwestern Indians and Mexicans. The Blackfoot cooked the roots and inhaled the steam for respiratory problems, while the Comanche used the leaves for whooping cough in a decoction. It was used by the Sioux for colds, coughs, and vertigo. Others used fresh flowers or roots for diarrhea, as a bath for fever, as a poultice for sores, bruises, and rheumatism. The Navajo, who used it for headaches, cuts, applied it to bee stings and snake bites, used a decoction of the root for excruciating urination, stomachache, colds, fever, and advocated the expulsion of the placenta during childbirth, which was perhaps most used. It was used regularly in sweat lodges and sweat baths as an ingredient.

3.50 Buck Brush

It is formally named Ceanothus, a generic term for some fifty to sixty North American shrubs species. The genus is restricted to North America, with a few species in the eastern United States, southeast Canada & reaching as far south as Guatemala. The distribution center is in California. Ceanothus velutinus, one species, was known by many Native American tribes as the Red Root, used for cysts, fibroid tumors, infection, and mouth and throat complications. Today, the treatment of high blood pressure, including lymphatic blockages, has also been shown to be successful. For a diuretic to stimulate kidney activity, another called the Hummingbird Blossoms was used. To ease childbirth, Ceanothus Integerrimus was used by North American tribes. Ceanothus sanguineus, generally referred to as Buckbrush Chaparral, was used for the prevention and relief of inflamed tonsils, swollen lymph nodes, enlarged spleens, non-fibrous cysts, menstrual bleeds, nosebleeds, hemorrhoids, and ulcers. Poultices have been used in the treatment of burns, cuts and sores. California's Miwok Indians were considered to have made baskets from Ceanothus branches, and the plant was used as an alternative for black tea by early pioneers.

3.51 Buckthorn

Native to the subtropical Northern Hemisphere and temperate and even more locally to the subtropical Southern Hemisphere in parts of Africa and South America, they are a genus of small trees or shrubs Rhamnaceae family. For medicinal purposes, only buckthorn bark is used. Buckthorn, known since the 14th century, is primarily administered as a laxative and purgative. Obesity, rheumatism, hepatitis, headache, allergies, intestinal worms, and skin disorders such as acne, eczema, and psoriasis have also been treated along with liver protection.

3.52 Buckwheat

This plant is not a grain but contains a fruit seed, a great source of fiber, manganese, and magnesium. It is formally called Fagopyrum Esculentum. It has traditionally been used as both a vegetable and in herbal medicines, even though it tastes quite bitter. It has been used to reduce bleeding, cure diarrhea, dysentery, skin infections, and a wide variety of circulatory disorders and decrease blood pressure and improve blood vessels.

3.53 Buffaloberry

There are three species which are called Canada Buffaloberry, Silver Buffaloberry (Shepherdia Argentea), Round-leaf Buffaloberry Shepherdia Rotundifolia and Russet Buffaloberry (Shepherdia Canadensis,). It is formally known as Shepherdia. In northern and western North America, these tiny shrubs with bitter-tasting berries are found. Often known as Silverleaf, rabbitberry, blueberry, chaparral berry, soapberry, and soopolallie, it has long been used as food, medicine, and dye. The Russet Bufalloberry has the most uses of the three forms. It was used to develop "Indian Ice Cream," which was a frothy dessert consisting of hot water, buffaloberries and sugar. Other drinks, sauces, preserves, porridge, dry cakes and more were also used. Constipation, tuberculosis, arthritis, swelling, cuts, venereal disorders, stomach issues, fever, broken bones, sore eyes, asthma, mosquito bites, boils, gallstones, toothaches, headache, and gynecological complaints were treated with the parts of the plant and also the berries. Buffaloberries are edible but very sour, leaving the mouth a little dry afterward.

3.54 Burdocks

This plant is formally named Arctium Lappa and is a part of the family of sunflowers, and is also classified as Cocklebur or Bardana. While it originated in Eurasia, it has for centuries been embraced and used by Native

Americans. Its roots have traditionally been consumed as a vegetable worldwide and have many medical applications in the treatment of stomach disorders and breathing problems. Native American applications included the grinding of the roots and leaves for skin protection, including sores and ulcers, and the Cherokee, Micmac, Maliseet, Menominee and Chippewa tribes used it for the treatment of rheumatism. It was noticed that the Iroquois used the roots to help in circulation and to purify the blood. It was also used by the Potawatomi as a blood purifier and a general tonic in teas. The Indians have used it as fruit, drying the roots for adding soups and using the young leaves as greens. It is rich in chromium, copper, potassium, magnesium, thiamin, phosphorus, vitamin A and zinc. Burdock was also used by several tribes for ritual purposes.

3.55 Alfalfa

Alfalfa is officially known as Medicago Sativa. It is a flowering plant in the family of peas. Grown all over the globe, it has been used for centuries in herbal medicine. It is best known because it is rich in protein, calcium, other nutrients, B group vitamins, vitamin C, vitamin K and vitamin E to alleviate digestive disruptions. It was used by Native Americans to encourage blood clotting and cure jaundice. Today, it is used for various medical conditions, including arthritis, muscle issues, lowering blood sugar levels, bone strength and alleviating signs of menopause. Avoid alfalfa if you have an auto-immune condition, as these forms of disorders have been known to worsen.

3.56 American Licorice

It is native to North America, from central Canada south across the United States to California, Texas and Virginia, but absent from the southeastern states. It is officially known as Glycyrrhiza Lepidota and is also called wild licorice. Several Native American tribes have commonly used its roots in teas for the treatment of stomach aches, cough, chest pain, diarrhea, fever, and to speed up placenta delivery after childbirth. It is also used on swelling as a wash or poultice. As a cure for toothaches and sore throats, the chewed root is kept in the mouth. The mashed leaves are used on sores as a poultice.

3.57 American Mistletoe

This is a species of mistletoe, known simply as Phoradendron Leucarpum. It is native to the United States and Mexico. Eastern Mistletoe, Oak Mistletoe, Pacific Mistletoe, Hairy Mistletoe and Western Mistletoe are its common names. Another mistletoe species was used by druids in Europe about 1,500 years ago for convulsions, delirium, paranoia, neuralgia, and cardiac problems. Phoradendron was used in analogous forms by Native Americans for blood pressure, respiratory disorders, epilepsy, headache and abortions. The Cherokee developed tea ooze, which was used for bathing the head for headache, and lung conditions, such as tuberculosis. The Creek made a concoction. The root was also used by the Mendocino Indians to stop pregnancy. Some applications involved biting on the root for toothaches, rubbing the body for sore limbs and knees. It has also been used in ritual rites by several tribes. The plant is known to be poisonous and should be used cautiously.

3.58 Antelope Sage

This plant, formally known as Eriogonum Jamesii, is a wild buckwheat species. This is also known as James' Buckwheat. Native to Arizona, Colorado, Utah, Texas, New Mexico, Oklahoma, and Nebraska in southwestern North America, it was also used by Native Americans, such as the Navajo, as a contraceptive. During menstruation, the ladies will drink one cup of a decoction of the root. To relieve the discomfort of childbirth, a decoction of the whole plant was sometimes used, and the root was chewed or used as a cardiac medicine in teas, for stomach aches, and depression. Others developed a wash which was used for sore eyes.

3.59 Arnica

One species, called Arnica Montana, a member of the sunflower family, has been used as a topical cream or ointment for centuries by Europeans and Native Americans to soothe muscle aches, alleviate pain, treat sprains and bruises, and cure wounds. Since it has caused serious and often lethal poisoning, Arnica should not be taken internally.

3.60 Aspen

Aspen trees are native to cold areas. This covers the extreme northern parts of North America and continues south at high altitudes in the mountains. There are many types of Aspen trees, one of which is the Quaking Aspen used to treat fever, scurvy, cough, discomfort, and as an anti-inflammatory by both Native Americans and early settlers. Salicin, a drug like aspirin's active ingredient, is found in the inner bark of this tree.

3.61 Astragalus

Native to the temperate areas of the Northern Hemisphere, it is a large genus of around 3,000 species of herbs and small shrubs. Used in ancient Chinese and Native American remedies, dried roots have also been used to protect the body against illness in conjunction with other herbs. The prevention of colds, fever, infection, allergies, asthma, weakness, anemia, burns, heart and kidney failure, measles, stomach ulcers, and intestinal diseases is the traditional medicinal applications. It is also known to help protect the body from illnesses such as cancer and diabetes. It is also used to protect and support the immune system, reduce colds, lower blood pressure, cure diabetes, and protect the liver.

3.62 Mayapple

This plant is native to wooded areas of eastern North America, officially known as Podophyllum Peltatum, has gone by various other names, including American Mandrake, Indian Apple, Ground Lemon, Ducks Foot, Hog Apple, Racoon Berry, Umbrella Vine, Love Apple, and others. The ripened fruit is edible in moderate amounts, but the fruit is toxic when eaten in large quantities. Many of the other areas of the plant are toxic. Folklore surrounds the Mayapple. It was said to have been used as a poison by witches. It was assumed that the English form of this herb, named Manroot (mandrake), was alive and that its cries would drive a man permanently mad when pulled from the ground. Native Americans used the edible fruit widely, eating it raw, frying it or turning it into preserves, jellies, marmalades, and pies. They also used it externally to cure snakebite, warts, and certain skin disorders. They have even used it on their crops as an insecticide. Later, Mayapple was used in Carter's Little Liver Pills as an ingredient. This herb can only be used by professional herbalists because of its toxicity.

3.63 Milkweed

This plant, also identified as Common Silkweed, Common Milkweed, Cottonweed, Silkweed, Wild Cotton, Virginia-Silk, and Silky Swallowwort, is officially known as Asclepias Syriaca, named for its milky juice. Milkweed was used as a food and medicine and made strings, ropes, and coarse fabric. It can be poisonous if not prepared properly. Various indigenous groups from eastern and mid-western America have boiled and consumed the flower buds, young shoots, stems, immature fruits, and butterfly milkweed roots as a vegetable. As a food supply, the flower buds were steamed by Meskwaki tribe, which were edible but not considered very flavorful. An infusion wa drunk by the Cherokee of traditional Virgin's Bower (Clematis species) and milkweed root for backache. They also used the herb as a laxative, a dropsy antidote, and a root infusion for venereal diseases. A decoction was used as contraception by the Meskwaki and Mohawk; the Iroquois and Navajo to avoid complications after childbirth, and the Chippewa to produce postpartum milk flow. Other uses included gastrointestinal issues, female problems, chest pain, warts, ringworm, and bee stings.

Warning: Without adequate preparation, milkweed can be poisonous when ingested internally.

3.64 Native Hemlock

This is a kind of conifer tree in the family of pine, officially named Tsuga. Tsuga species are not toxic, unlike poisonous hemlock (conium). It was also used as a dye for tanning skins, producing baskets & wooden products by area tribes. As a poultice or salve for colds and to avoid sunburn, the pitch was also added topically. Pounded bark decoctions were also used for the prevention of hemorrhages. Native Americans have used another species, usually referred to as the Mountain Hemlock (Tsuga Mertensiana). The inner bark and twigs in a tea were used by the Menominee and the Woodland Potawatomi to treat colds and fever. It was sometimes used to cure fever, kidney or bowel complications, pneumonia, as a gargle for problems with the mouth and throat, and to wash sores and ulcers externally.

3.65 The Oak

These trees and shrubs are scientifically called Quercus and have over 600 species distributed all over the world. Its fruit, the acorn, was a favorite in many Native American cultures, and for several ailments, the tree's inner bark was used. Acorns are an excellent diet for those suffering from degenerative, wasting diseases like tuberculosis. To produce a bitter decoction used in the treatment of diarrhea gargles for sore throats, kidney and urinary disorders, viruses, and menstrual bleeding, Native Americans used the oak's inner bark. Poultices were effectively utilized for treating ringworm, wounds, sores, sprains, and swelling.

3.66 Osha

It is also called Porter's Licorice Root, Colorado Cough Root, Osha Root, Bear Root, and is officially known as Ligusticum Porteri. It is called Bear Root & Bear Medicine in certain Native American cultures. In the celery family, this aromatic plant grows in the Southwest in the desert woodlands.

The whole plant was used medicinally, but the most widely regarded are the thick taproots. It was widely traded by Native Americans with a wide range of medicinal properties and highly regarded, so tribes far away from the ancestral plants still used the herb in the ceremonies and medicines. In teas, tonics, and chewed for internal use, Osha roots, either fresh or dry, are made into poultices and salves for external use. Warming properties have been used for cold and chills and to promote circulation. Salves and liniments were used by the Apache and Indians as snake and mosquito repellent because of the strong smell. It was also used for sore joints, body aches, rheumatism, and arthritis. It has been used internally for stomach issues, breathing problems, headache, flu and cold systems, fever, sinusitis, and heartburn. The Osha root has also been used by several tribes as incense during ceremonies. The Chiricahua and Mescalero Apache use the herbal root with chilies as a culinary seasoning for flavoring beef.

3.67 Partridgeberry

It is native to America, formally named Mitchella Repens, and is also known by some common names like One-berry, Deerberry, Squaw Vine, and Winter Clover. Partridgeberry had extra used for Native American tribes, including ritual smoke, a love potion, and snack when the berries were ingested or used in sauces, bread, and cakes, while mainly used in medicines.

Many Native Americans, like the Cherokee, made tea from the boiled leaves that were consumed to relieve labor during the final weeks of pregnancy. A lotion made from the leaves was applied to their breasts by nursing mothers to alleviate soreness. The tea was also used by early colonists as a breastfeeding aid and as a cure for menstrual cramps. It has also been used to relieve pains and cramps in menstruation, monitor menstruation, and induce childbirth. As an abortifacient, it can also be effective and should not be used by pregnant women.

3.68 Passionflower

It is also generally regarded as Passion Vine, formally named Passiflora. It is distributed across the world, comprising 500 species of flowering plants, but nine species are native to the USA. One plant has a long history of usage by Native Americans, usually called Maypop, and was adapted by early European colonists. To cure insomnia, anxiety, paranoia, delusions, and epilepsy, the leaves and roots were used to produce a drink. It was also used to prevent depression, hyperactivity, tension, muscle pain, and burns, cuts, boils, and ear pain in poultices. If you are pregnant or breastfeeding, do not take the passionflower.

3.69 Pau d'arco

This plant, native to South America, is scientifically known as Tabebuia Avellanedae and is used to treat a wide variety of conditions. It has historically been used to relieve pain, arthritis, prostate gland inflammation, fever, dysentery, ulcers and boils, and various cancers.

3.70 Pennyroyal

This part of the Mint family is scientifically named Mentha Pulegium and has long been used as a culinary herb & folk remedy. It was widely used by the Greeks and Romans as a cooking plant, and it was also used by the Greeks in wine production. Mock Pennyroyal, Mosquito Vine, Fleabane, Tickweed, and Stinking Balm are sometimes called American Pennyroyal. It was used in colonial America to eradicate rodents, including snakes. While it is believed to be poisonous, Native Americans have used American Pennyroyal widely to relieve headache, watery eyes, stomach aches, itching, fever and induce menstrual discharge. The leaves were externally crushed and applied to the skin as an insect repellant. It has also been used as an abortifacient for preventing flatulence, hepatitis, gall disease, gout, gums, and tumors. Pennyroyal is not meant to be used by pregnant women in any way. Death has been caused by overconsumption of this plant.

3.71 Pinon

This member of the Pine genus, formally named Penus Edulis, is native to the U.S. and is present in southern Wyoming, Colorado, northern Arizona, New Mexico, eastern and central Utah, and westernmost Texas in the Guadalupe Mountains. Native Americans gathered the pine nuts and edible seeds widely, with some tribes referring to it as the "tree of life." In addition to using the tree for fruit and wood, the Mescalero Apache, and the Navajo in their Evilway ritual often used it for religious reasons such as girls' puberty rites. It has been used to cure colds for medical purposes by inhaling smoke from needles.

For various medical uses, including swallowing the needles or using them in an infusion, the Zuni used the piñon to facilitate sweating. For skin infections, bruises, and sores, and as an antiseptic, they even ground the resin. By blending the piñon pitch with whisky and brown sugar, the Spanish New Mexicans handled the same illness.

3.72 The Plantain

It also has many other common names, scientifically named Waybread, Snakeweed, Plantago Major, including Ripple Grass, Cuckoo's Bread, Englishman's Foot, White Man's Foot, among others. It was known by the ancient Saxon people to be one of the nine holy herbs and has a long tradition of usage as an alternative medicine dating back to ancient times. More than 200 species are native to northern and central Asia and Europe. As one of their favorite medicinal treatments, early colonists introduced plantain to North America, and it was quickly named White Man's Foot by Native Americans, as it is frequently seen rising along well-trodden footpaths. Many of the typical European uses for this beneficial herb were rapidly embraced by Native Americans. For a variety of treatments, the seeds and leaves were used to remove rattlesnake bite venom, soothe rheumatic discomfort, as a poultice to relieve fighting wounds, sores, bug bites, tuberculosis, bronchitis, laryngitis, sore throat, urinary diseases, stomach issues, and a tonic that purifies the blood. To alleviate toothache, the root of the herb was used, and the juice to relieve ear pain.

3.73 Pleurisy Root

This is a genus of milkweed native to eastern North America, also known by many other names, like Flux Root, Swallowwort, Butterfly Weed, Canada Root, Tuber Root, White Root, Wind Root and Orange. Due to its potential to reduce inflammation, it has long been considered an important therapy for many respiratory disorders. It has been used to treat cough, pleurisy (inflammation of the lungs), pneumonia, uterine conditions, pain, spasms, flu, bronchitis, alleviate respiration, and facilitate sweating. It was reported that the Natchez tribes drank tea from the boiling roots as a cure for pneumonia and to facilitate the removal of phlegm.

Poke

This perennial herb is scientifically known as Phytolacca Americana and is a native weed of the eastern United States. Many other names are common, like American Nightshade, Poke Grass, Inkberry, Pigeon Berry, Redweed, Pocan Bush, and others. While parts of this plant are highly poisonous to livestock and humans, and farmers consider it a major pest, certain parts of the plant have been used for food and medicine for a long time. It has traditionally been used to cure syphilis, diphtheria, cancer, intestinal worms, cramps, hypertension, stomach ulcers to strengthen the reproductive, urinary, and immune systems. Skin disorders, inflammation, rheumatism, abscesses, swelling, discomfort, sprains, and hemorrhoids were used with poultices and washes.

3.74 Prickly Pear Cactus

This plant has the significance of being a vegetable, fruit, and herb, scientifically known as Opuntia Engelmanni, which has been used both for food and medicine. It is also known by many common names, including Texas Prickly Pear, Cow's Tongue Cactus, Desert Prickly Pear, among others, and is common in the Southwestern United States and northern Mexico. The younger pads were used by Native Americans for food, and mature pads were used as a poultice for cuts, burns, boils, bleeding slows, enlarged prostate, and as an antiseptic. Teas have been developed internally to cure tuberculosis, urinary tract infections and the immune system. Cholesterol reduction and the treatment of diet-related cardiovascular disease and adult-onset diabetes may also be treated effectively with this herb.

3.75 AmericanSpikenard

Due to its aromatic roots, it is strongly linked to wild sarsaparilla. To have therapeutic purposes, any portion of this herb has been used in every way: curing angina, back pain, earaches, skin infections, preventing cough & premenstrual syndrome.

3.76 Blazing Star

This plant was used by American Indians as a means of food and medicine. Used for the reduction of swelling, stomach pain and snake bite antidote.

3.77 California Poppy

It was used to treat aches, insomnia and agitation. It was also widely used to treat bed wetting among children.

Coneflower- Purple and Yellow

This herb has immune-stimulant and anti-inflammatory properties. The Indians used it effectively to treat colds and coughs.

3.78 Hyssop

For intestinal inflammation, bronchitis and respiratory diseases, urinary tract infection, sore throat, coughs, asthma, flatulence and colic, and sedative effects, hyssop was used orally as a drink. Hyssop is used topically in baths to cause sweating; and for treating skin irritations, wounds.

3.79 Indian Tobacco

The plant root is used to cure leg ulcers, abscesses, and bronchodilators for asthma and whooping cough. It reduces nicotine withdrawal effects.

3.80 Turtlehead

The turtlehead plant is usually made into a tonic or leaf tea and is used as a gentle laxative and the ability to remove worms. It has also been used to increase appetite and improve the function of the stomach and liver.

The leaves and stems are ground to be used externally on sores and fever blisters and made into an ointment or poultice. It helps control blood pressure and for the health of the liver.

3.81 Yellow Spined Thistle

It is scientifically called Cirsium Ochrocentrum. It is native to the central United States. It has been used in herbal treatments for a long time by Native Americans. It has been used for many purposes by the Zuni people, including contraception and curing syphilis and diabetes. The Kiowa also used the plant for wounds, sores, and other skin disorders as a wash.

3.82 Yerba Mate

Officially named Ilex Paraguariensis, Holly's genus is sometimes spelled Erva Mate and is a species of Holly. It is native to subtropical South America. As a therapeutic herb used for anything from raising immunity and purifying the blood to reducing depression and curing insomnia, it has a long history.

It has also been used to alleviate exhaustion, curb hunger, cure stomach and intestinal issues, lower blood pressure, detoxify the body, nervous discomfort, depression, anxiety, fever, obesity, and strengthen the nervous and muscle systems a diuretic, tonic and as a stimulant.

3.83 Yellow dock

This widespread weed from the Buckwheat family is naturalized in North America, officially known as Rumex Crispus. Often known as Sour Dock, Curly Dock and

Narrow Dock, it was soon adopted as a common medicine and food by Native Americans. Different cultures throughout North America have used both the leaves and roots to cure constipation, ringworm, purify the blood and stomach aches. It has been used externally for joint discomfort, swelling, mild sores, diaper rash, and other scalp irritations. The Navajo used the root as a tonic, calling it a "life medicine" and a warm wash made from the decoction of crushed roots for a disinfectant recommended by Cherokee herbalists.

3.84 Yellow Root

Officially named Xanthorhiza Simplicissima, from Maine south to northern Florida and west to Ohio and eastern Texas, this woody-stemmed plant is native to the eastern United States. Although Yellow Root is poisonous in large quantities, for treatment of mouth disorders, stomach ulcers, stomach ache, Native Americans made a tea and used it externally on skin conditions, sores and swelling. It has also been shown to be effective for reducing blood pressure and the liver's well-being.

3.85 Witch Hazel

It is made from the bark and leaves the North American Witch-hazel shrub, known officially as Hamamelis Virginiana, a proven astringent. It grows naturally in the

United States from Nova Scotia west to Ontario, Canada, and south to Florida and Texas and has been extensively used by American Indians for medicinal purposes. By boiling the shrub stems, the Witch Hazel extract was developed to cure sore muscles, wounds, bug bites, skin irritations, sores, bruising, swelling, and to avoid bleeding. The Wisconsin Menominee heated the leaves and rubbed the substance on the legs of tribesmen interested in sports games. A decoction of the boiled twigs was used to relieve aching backs, while a favorite Potawatomi remedy for muscle aches was steam obtained from dropping the twigs in water with hot rocks. This cure was adopted from the natives by early Puritan settlers in New England, and its use became generally known in the United States. In the prevention of acne, eczema, psoriasis, ingrown nails, broken or blistered lips, poison ivy, hemorrhoids, varicose veins, and sunburn, it has also been shown to be effective. While witch hazel has been used by eastern American Indians to treat several ailments, the Chippewa used it primarily to treat swollen, inflamed, or irritated eyes.

3.86 Wild Onion

About 600 onion species (Allium) are found in North America, Europe, Northern Africa, and Asia. Moreover, chives, shallots, leeks, and garlic also form part of the onion family. Hey may be used as ornamentals, vegetables, and spices. These are used to treat colds, coughs, allergies, lung infections, bronchitis, and insect repellent.

Willow

There are approximately 400 species of trees and shrubs. The leaves and bark of the willow tree have been alluded to for aches and fever in ancient texts from Egypt and Greece. It was relied on by Native Americans throughout the American continent as a cornerstone in their medical care. It is because willows contain Salicin, which is a substance that resembles aspirin chemically. It was also used to treat nausea, headache, mouth sores, toothache, diarrhea trouble with the stomach. The Pomo tribe also boiled the root bark’s inner part for tea use in chills and fever cases to cause sweating. From the red willow's bark, the Natchez prepared their fever treatments in the south, whereas the Alabama and Creek Indians plunged for the same reason into willow root baths.

Wild Ginger

It is also known as Canada Wild Ginger and Canadian Snakeroot, formally known as Asarum Canadense, and is native to eastern North America forests. In the treatment of dysentery, stomach issues, swollen breasts, cough and colds, sore throat, typhus, scarlet fever, nerves, cramps, earache, hypertension, measles, headache, convulsions, urinary diseases and venereal disease, Native Americans used the roots as a spice as well as an herbal plant. They also used it as an appetite enhancer.

Lettuce

It is also named Opium Lettuce, Green Endive, and Acrid Lettuce, formally known as Lactuca Virosa. It was used for sedative purposes, especially in nervous complaints, and was native to North America. The health benefits of wild lettuce tea have been well established, and some of this herb's medicinal acts are mentioned in ancient Egyptian writings and artwork. It has been used for the treatment of colic, insomnia, anxiety, stress, and cough.

Wild Black Cherry

It is also known as Mountain Black Cherry, Black Cherry, Rum Cherry, Black Choke, Choke Cherry. It is officially known as Prunus Serotina. From eastern Canada to southern Quebec and Ontario, it is native to eastern North America. The dried inner bark was historically used for cough, whooping cough, blood tonic, fever, cold, measles, bronchitis, laryngitis, cough, sore throat, asthma, elevated blood pressure, colic, arthritis, edema, diarrhea, lung disease, inflammation of the skin, swelling lymph glands, pneumonia, tuberculosis, diseases of autoimmune fever, and dyspepsia in tea or syrup. It was often considered useful for impaired breathing, loss of appetite, and moderate sedative. The Mohegan tribe used it to treat dysentery, and it was believed that the Meskwaki tribe had made a root bark's sedative tea. Remember that the seeds and leaves are venomous.

White pine

Officially known as PinuIs Strobus, and commonly known as Deal Pine and Soft Pine.

It is native to North America. Native Americans have long used the inner bark, young shoots, twigs, pitch, and leaves in herbal treatments to cure colds, cough, measles, pneumonia, fever, heartburn, headache, inflammation, neuritis, bronchitis, croup, laryngitis, and kidney complications. The inner bark or sap as a poultice for wounds and sores by some Native American tribes. Pitch has been used for "drawing out" boils, splinters, abscesses, and for rheumatism, broken bones, cuts, bruising, and inflammation as well. Sometimes on a hot cloth, a hot resin was spread and applied to relieve pneumonia, sciatic pain, and general muscle pain.

Western Skunk Cabbage

It is sometimes called Yellow Skunk Cabbage or Swamp Lantern, formally referred to as Lysichiton Americanus.

Found in the Pacific Northeast in swamps and damp forests, it has a "skunky" scent that permeates the region where the plant grows. The plant was used by Native Americans as a drug for wounds and bruises and to treat sores and swelling. It was also used in times of drought as bread. The flavor of the leaves is very acidic or peppery. However, since it contains calcium oxalate crystals, it is not advised that the cabbage be eaten, which produces a sharp prickling feeling on the tongue and throat, resulting in digestive inflammation and even death if consumed in sufficient amounts.

Conclusion

Ever since ancient times, people from all continents have been using thousands of indigenous plants to cure illnesses. These ancient peoples, by watching animals, studied what herbs and plants would fit with different situations. The use of plants for medicines predates written human history, but the oldest archaeological evidence suggests that a 60,000-year-old burial site in Neanderthal developed significant pollen quantities from plants that were later believed to have been used in herbal remedies. For the Sumerians, who identified well-established medicinal uses for plants like laurel, caraway and thyme, the historical evidence on herbs dates back over 5,000 years. Ancient Egyptian medicine used castor oil, mint, garlic, opium, coriander, indigo and other plants for curing various illnesses. Herb use and cultivation of plants like vetch, mandrake, caraway, wheat, barley and rye are also mentioned in the Old Testament of the Bible. Herbalism is also identified using herbs, plant extracts, minerals, fungal and animal products and shells. Currently, pills, capsules, powders, teas, extracts and new or dried plants contain herbs. Many of these may be very helpful; but, when using any of these strong supplements, care should be taken. Some, when they interfere with other medicines, can cause health problems. Before taking herbal supplements, it is advised to contact the doctor, please follow the guidelines on the label, and be very cautious if you are pregnant or breastfeeding. Some separation of infectious disease has been practiced by most Native North Americans, normally by sending the patient to a location far away from the tribe. During an outbreak, the healthier participants may often isolate themselves from a distance. Braves injured in battle were generally separated until they were recovered from the tribe. It was commonly used to provide a sweat bath or vapor bath. Initially, with extended exposure to dry heat, it was comparable to a Finnish sauna, accompanied perhaps by water tossed on to the hot stones. It was supposedly used for general hygiene (e.g., the Native Americans of the Hudson River), for joint pain management (the Saponas) or with the use of medicinal herbs (the Choctaws). As part of the holistic treatment regime, the physical cleansing in the sweat lodge was also followed by religious rituals. Early visitors reflected positively on the tribes' high levels of personal grooming and their villages' cleanliness. Although many of the Native North American remedies were accepted as ethical medicines, patent medicine was also emerging. Tuscarora Rice, named after an Iroquois tribe and sold as a treatment for tuberculosis, was the first North American patent medicine (1711). A wave of patent medicines followed this, often with the term "Indian" on the label to signify an aboriginal origin, although the ingredients may have originated from abroad. Several oral preparations were strong in alcohol, offering an instant feeling of wellbeing. Medicine shows became the predecessors of today's soap operas. A mini-circus, conducting war dances, and offering riding exhibitions and other shows were employed to tour native North Americans. This pulled in the fans and their "commercials," the hard-selling of so-called "genuine native remedies. These shows existed between the Civil War and the World War of 1914-18 (1856-1917), but only a few survived the World War of 1939-45. Native American medicine is focused on traditional ideas of healthy living, the consequences of disease-producing actions, and the moral ideals that restore stability. Both tribes hold these beliefs; however, the techniques of diagnosis and care differ considerably from tribe to tribe and healer to healer. Anyone who truly desires to live a life of wholeness and balance may benefit from Native American medicine. Those benefits can be physical, mental, or spiritual. There is, nevertheless, the understanding that the white man's diseases or "the diseases of civilization," do require the white man's medicine. Native American medicine may be an important aspect of an integrative approach to treatment in these situations. Faith's role in the healing process is the main distinction between Native American healing and traditional medicine, both in the past and present. Native Americans claim that all things in nature are connected and that spirits may foster wellbeing or induce illness. Thus, not just the physical aspects of a person, but both their mental wellbeing and emotional wellbeing must be healed.

CPSIA information can be obtained
at www.ICGtesting.com
Printed in the USA
LVHW020545090621
689685LV00003B/95

9 781802 350630